Recipe Name

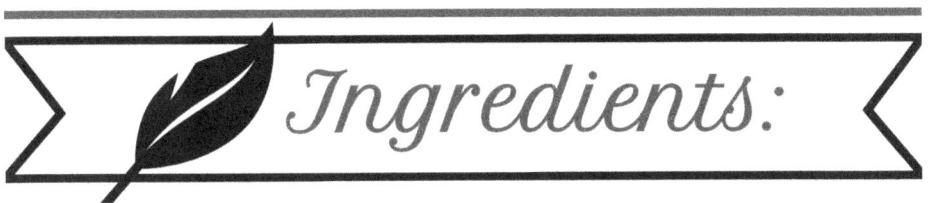

Ingredients:

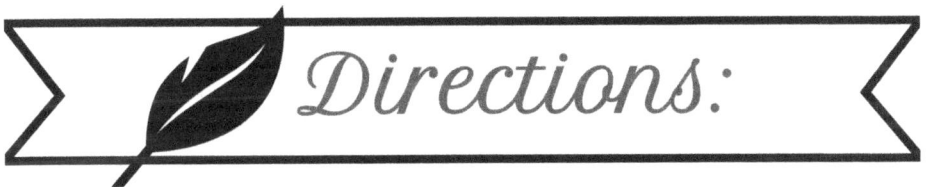

Directions:

Recipe Name

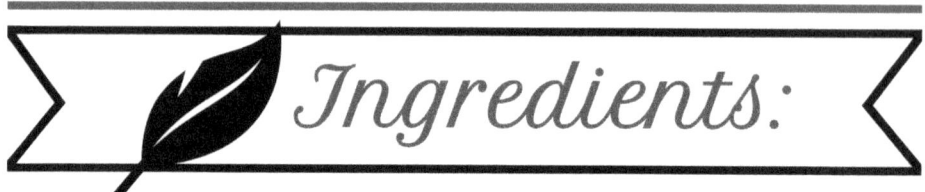

Ingredients:

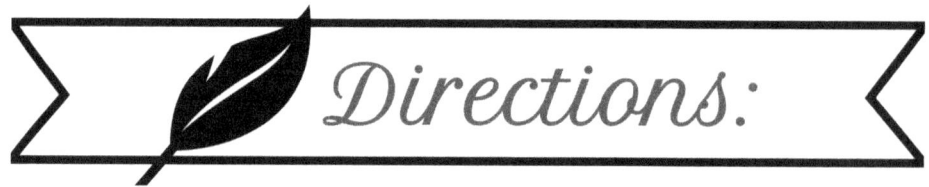

Directions:

Recipe Name

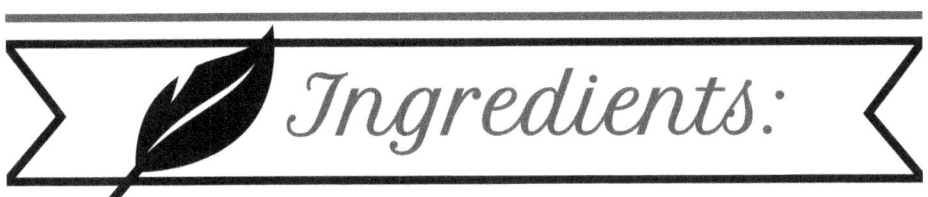

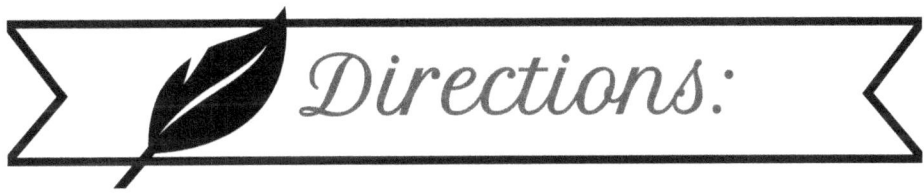

Recipe Name

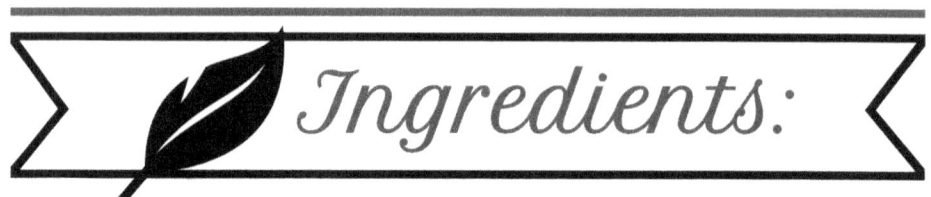

Ingredients:

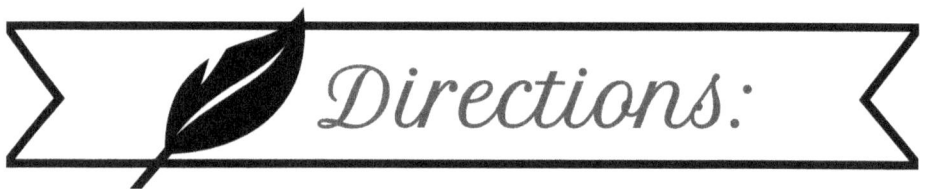

Directions:

Recipe Name

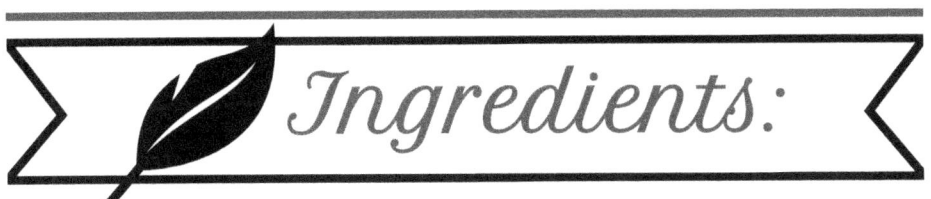

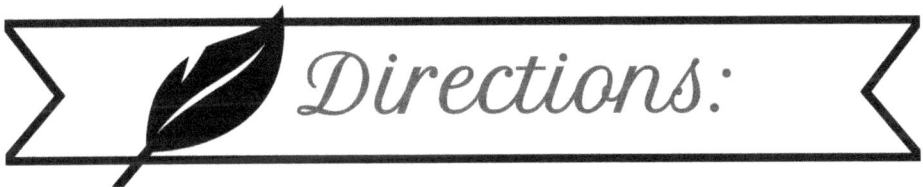

Recipe Name

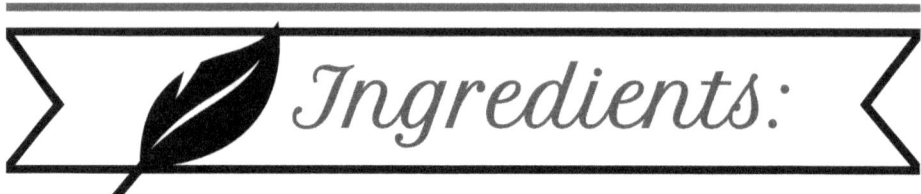

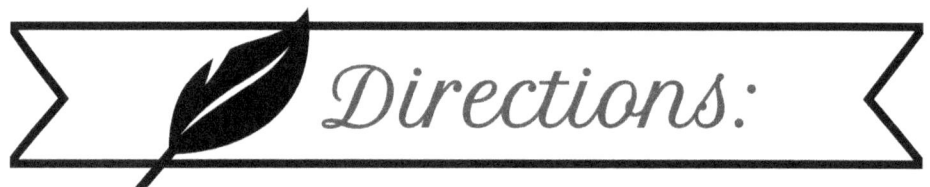

Recipe Name

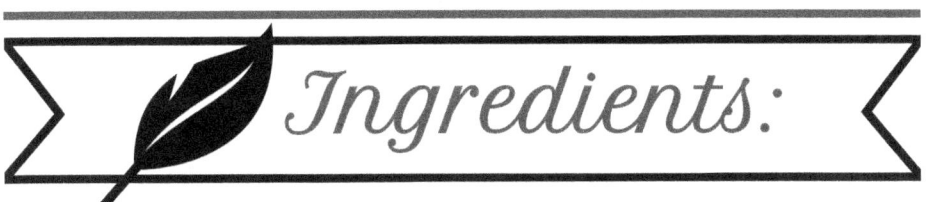

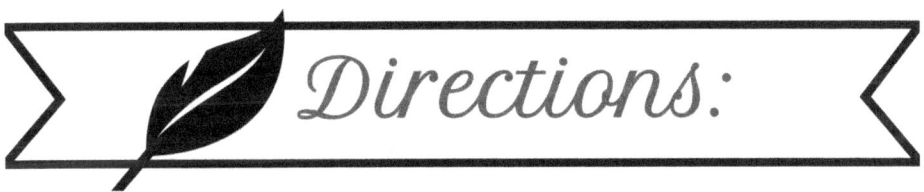

Recipe Name

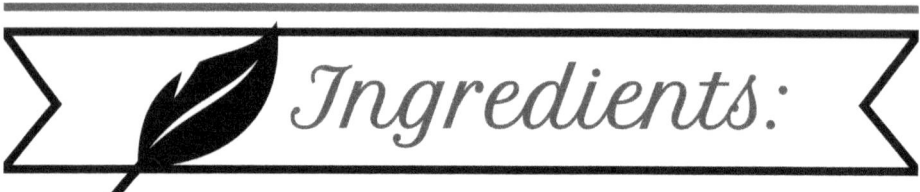

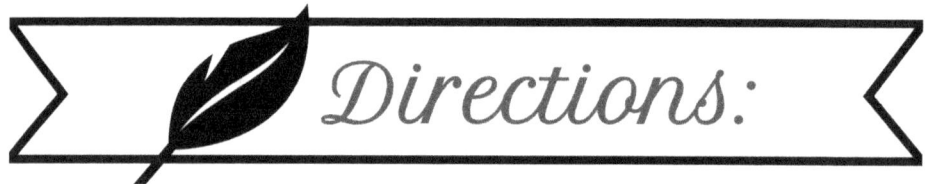

Recipe Name

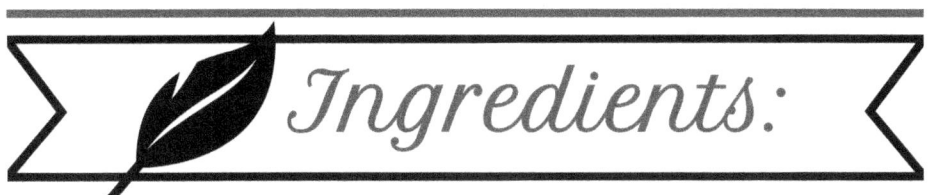

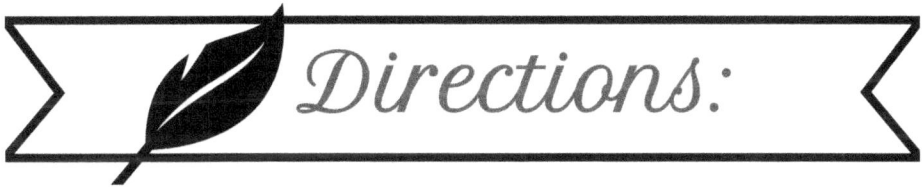

Recipe Name

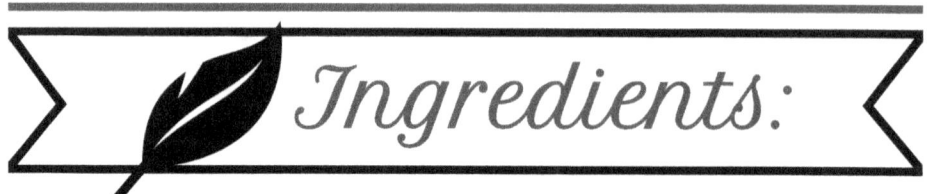

Ingredients:

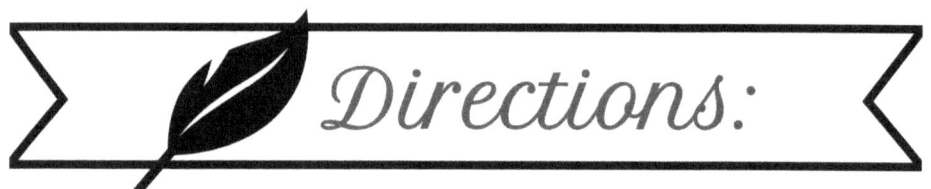

Directions:

Recipe Name

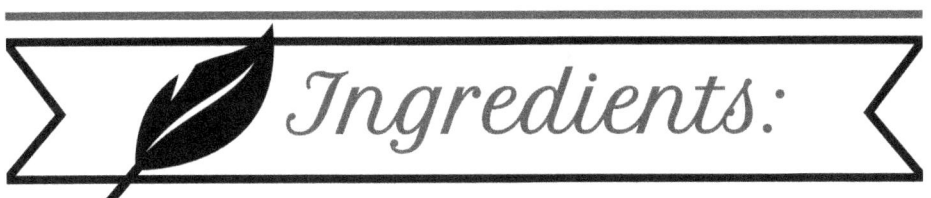

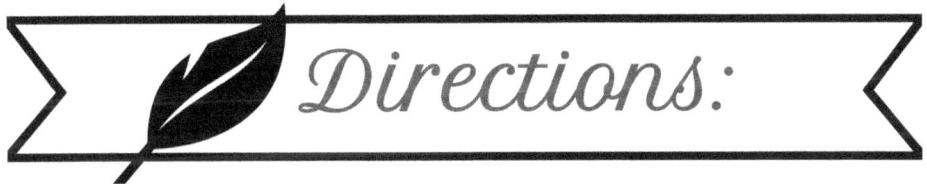

Recipe Name

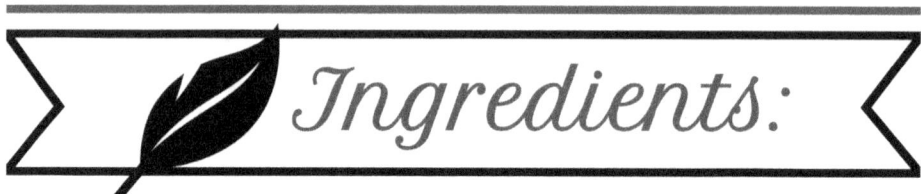

Ingredients:

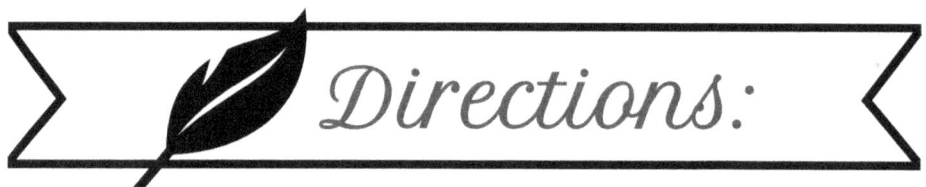

Directions:

Recipe Name

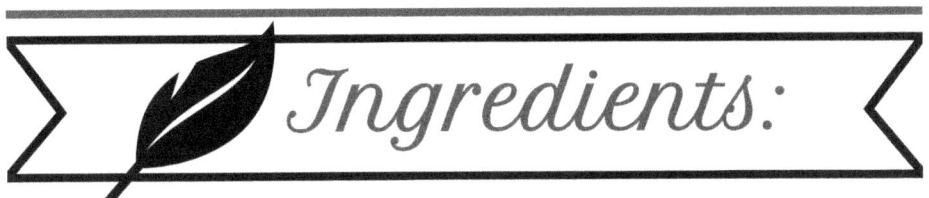

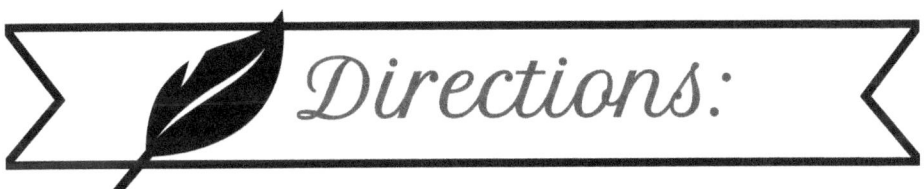

Recipe Name

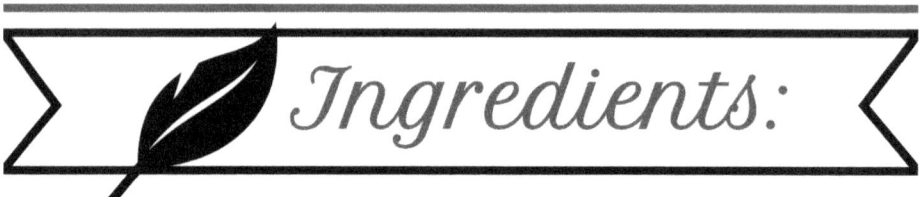

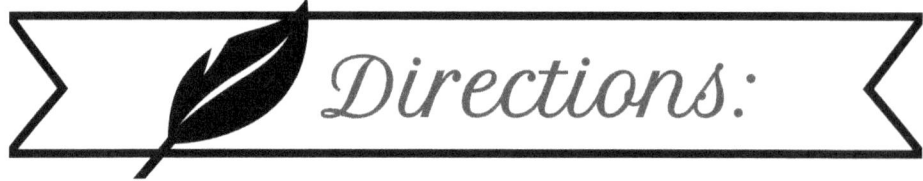

Recipe Name

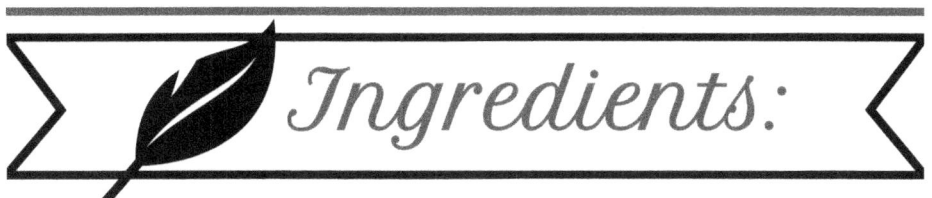

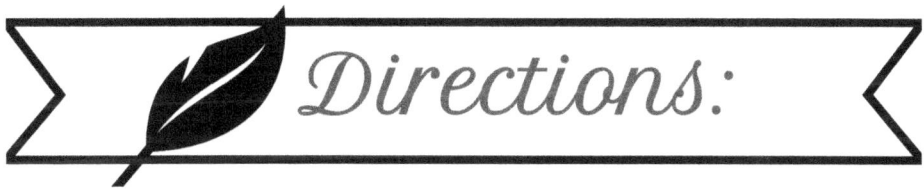

Recipe Name

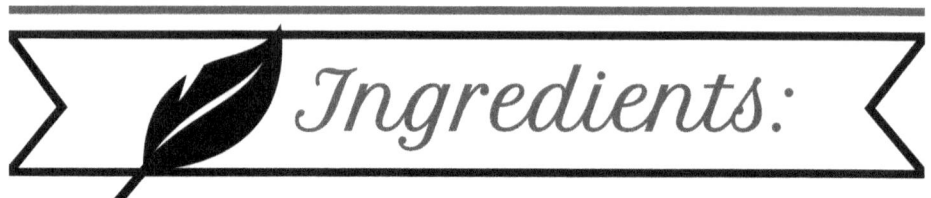

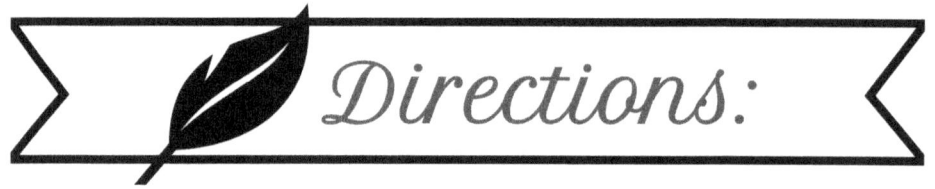

Recipe Name

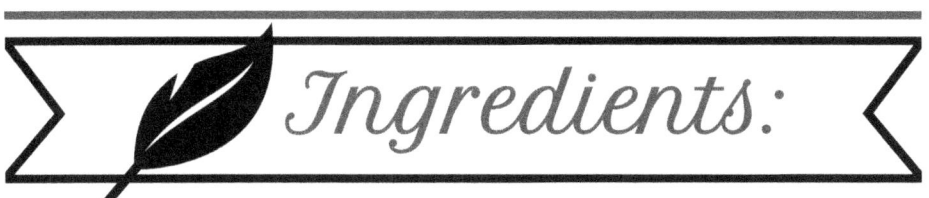

Ingredients:

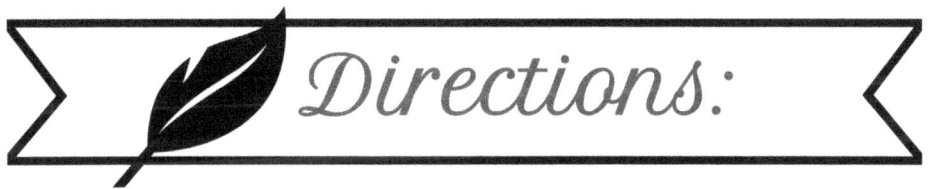

Directions:

Recipe Name

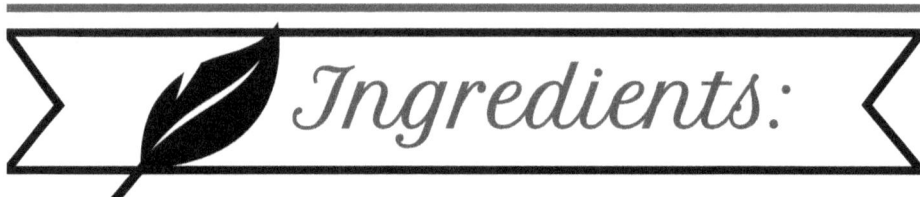

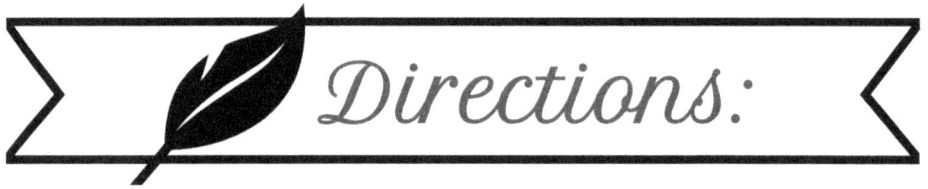

Recipe Name

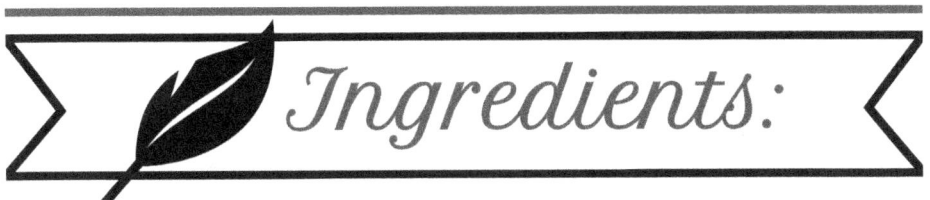

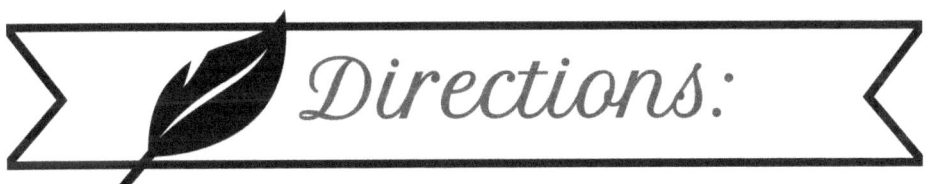

Recipe Name

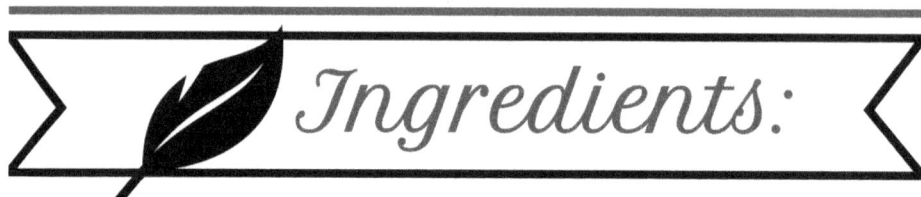

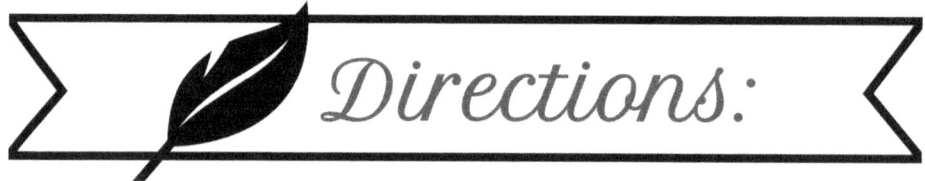

Recipe Name

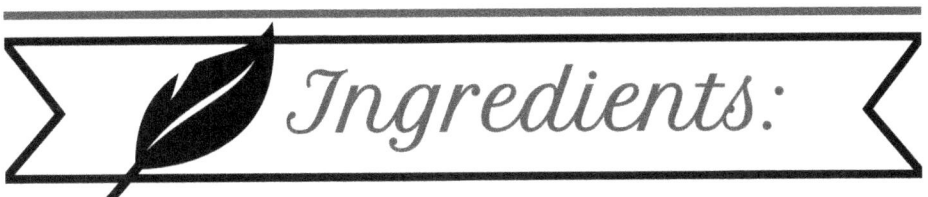

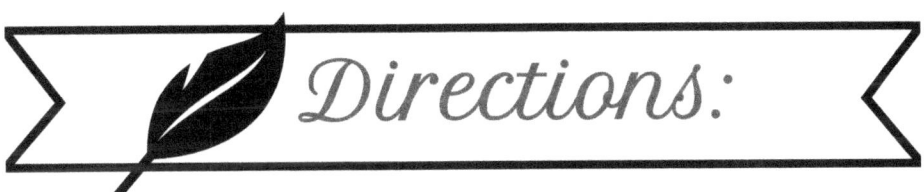

Recipe Name

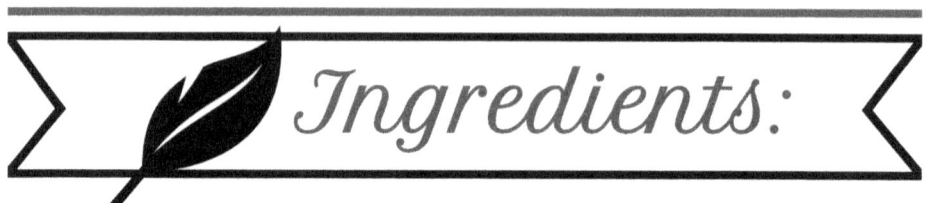

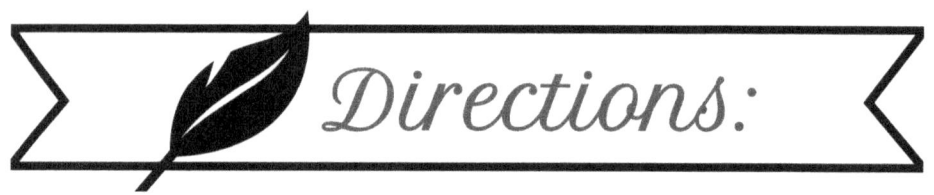

Recipe Name

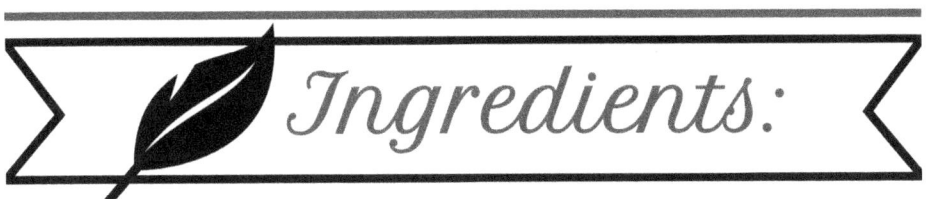

Ingredients:

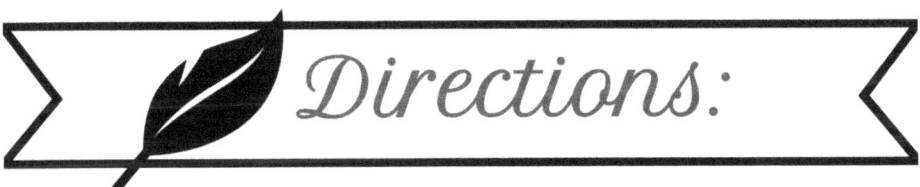

Directions:

Recipe Name

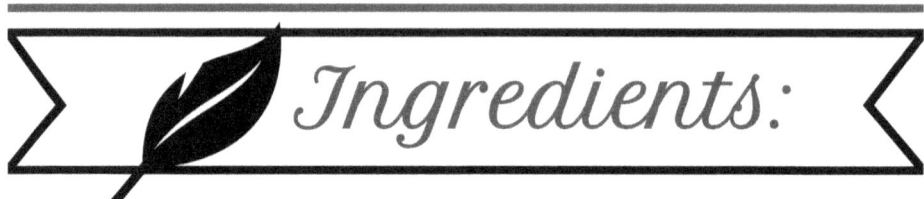

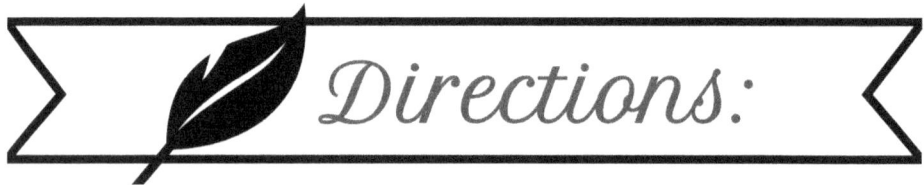

Recipe Name

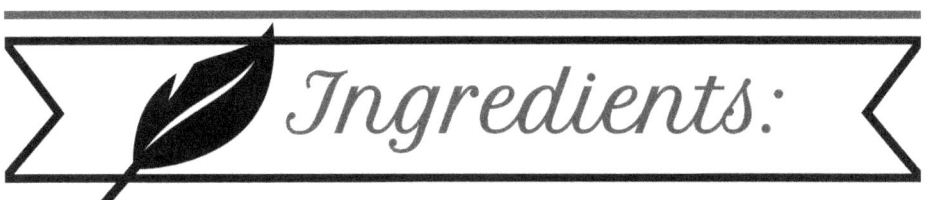

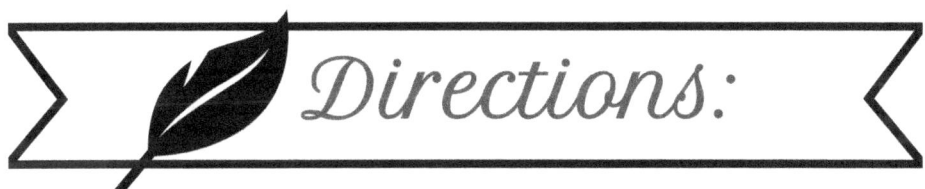

Recipe Name

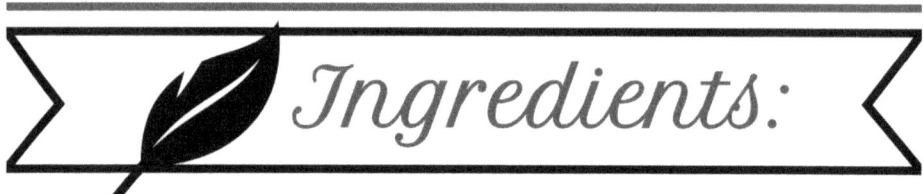

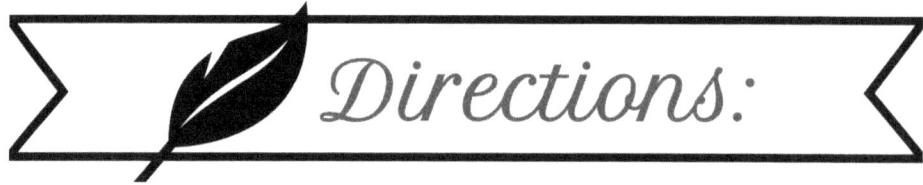

Recipe Name

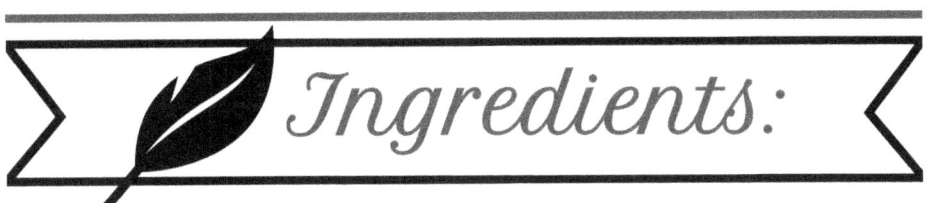

Ingredients:

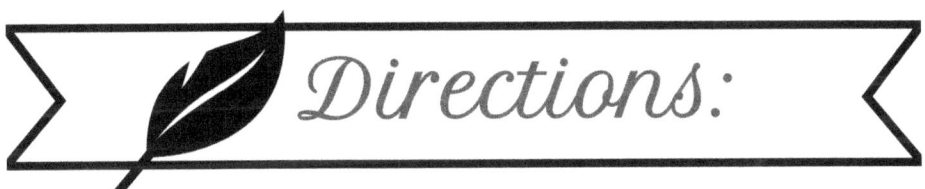

Directions:

Recipe Name

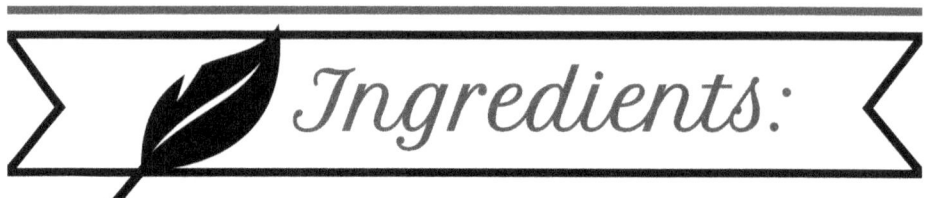

Ingredients:

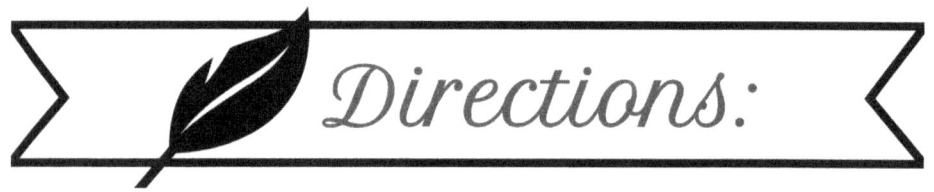

Directions:

Recipe Name

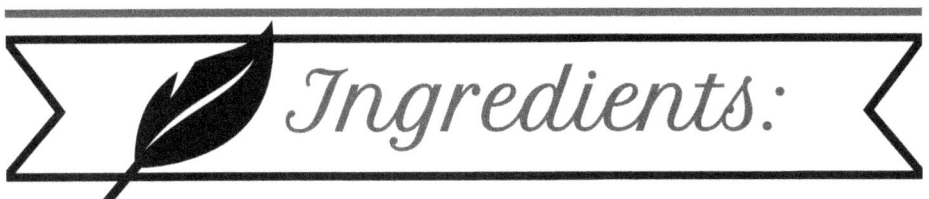

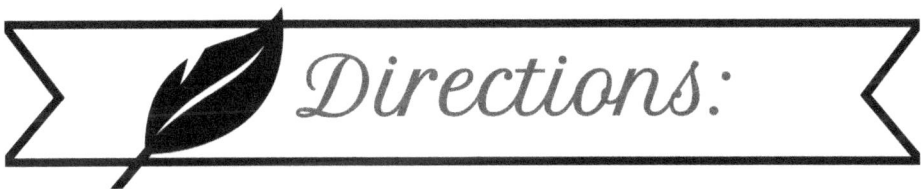

Recipe Name

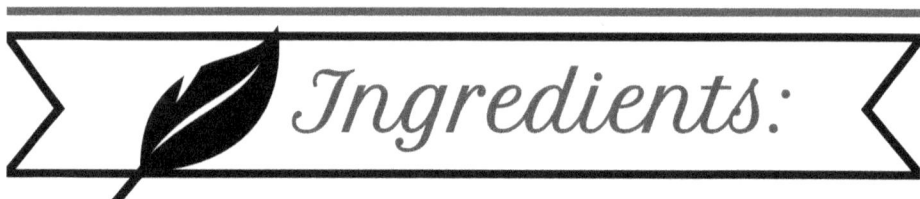

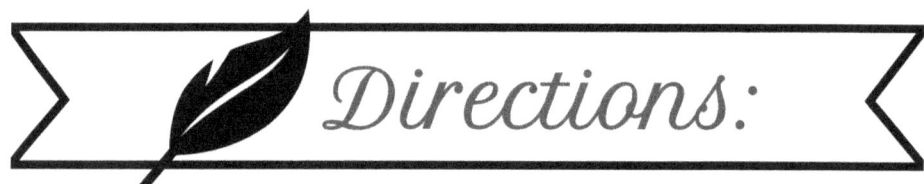

Recipe Name

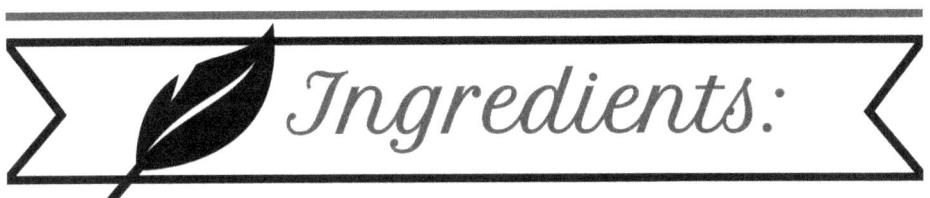

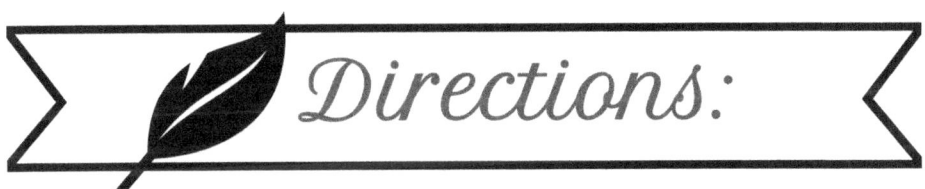

Recipe Name

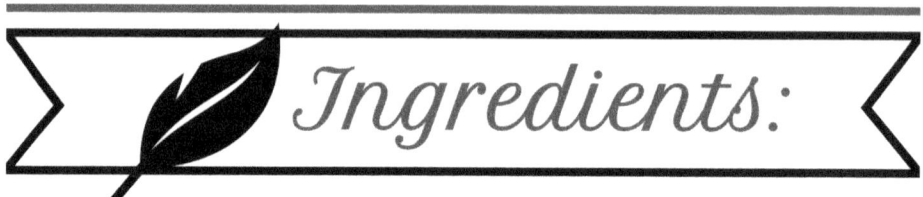

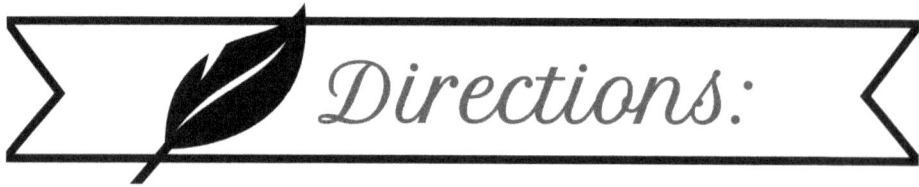

Recipe Name

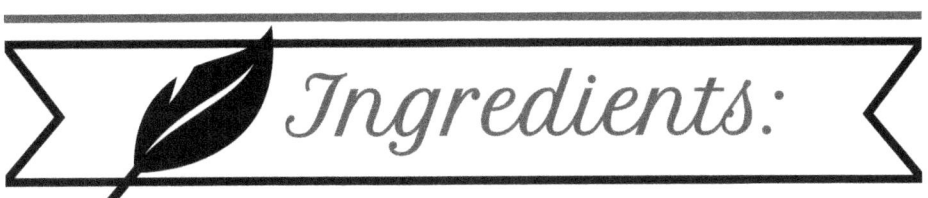

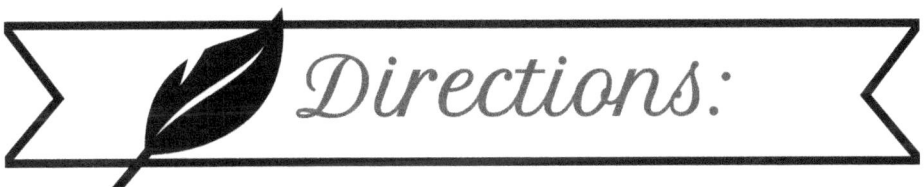

Recipe Name

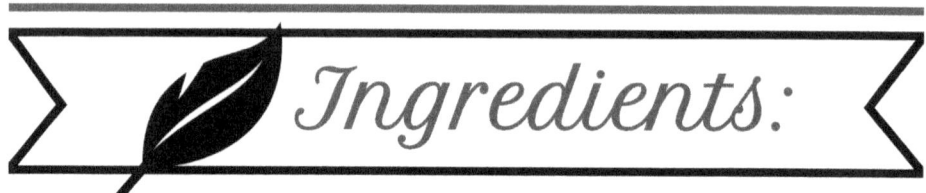

Ingredients:

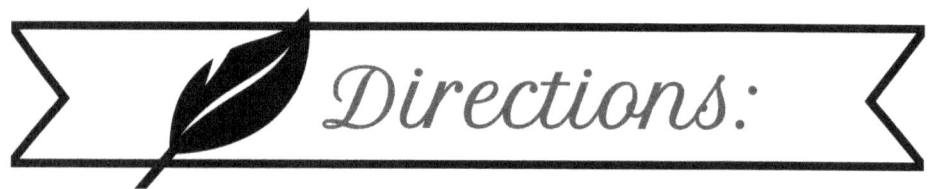

Directions:

Recipe Name

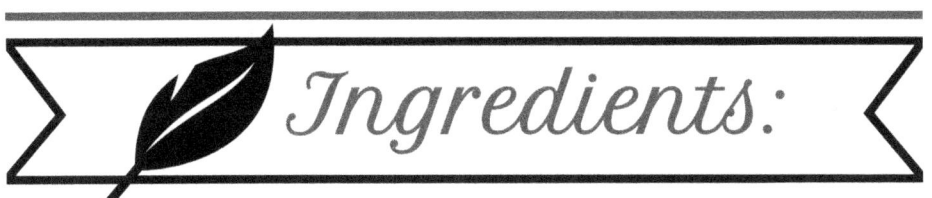

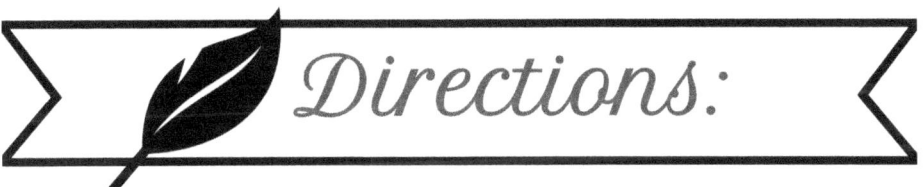

Recipe Name

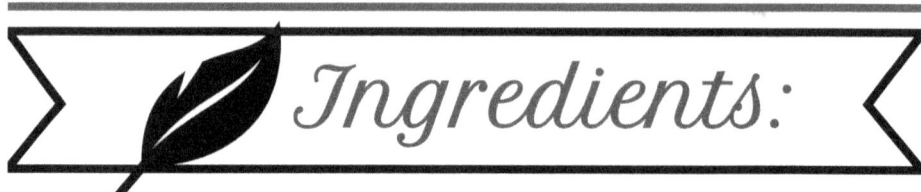

Ingredients:

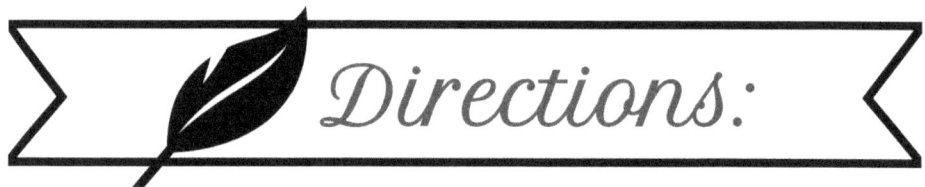

Directions:

Recipe Name

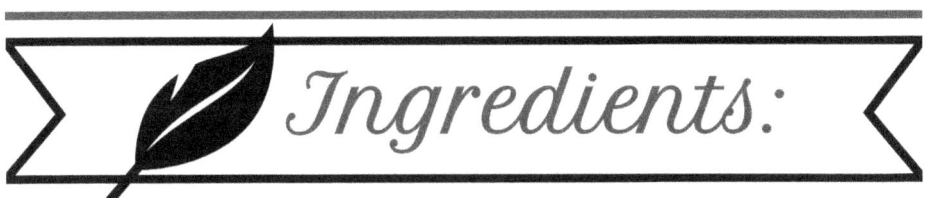

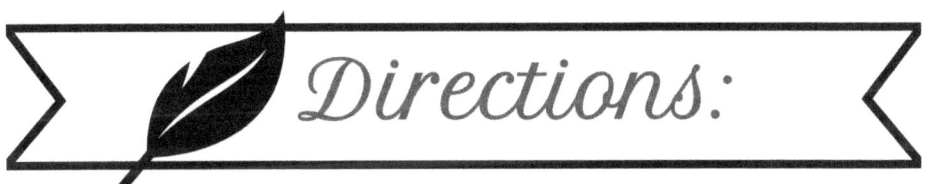

Recipe Name

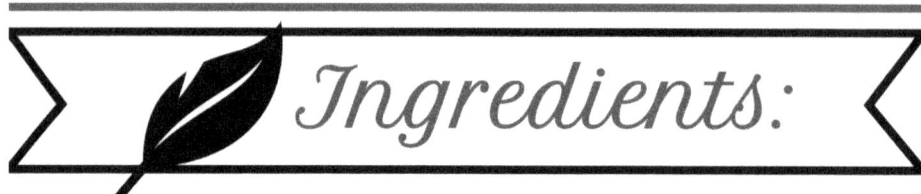

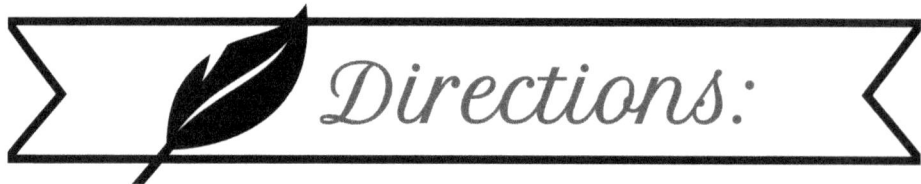

Recipe Name

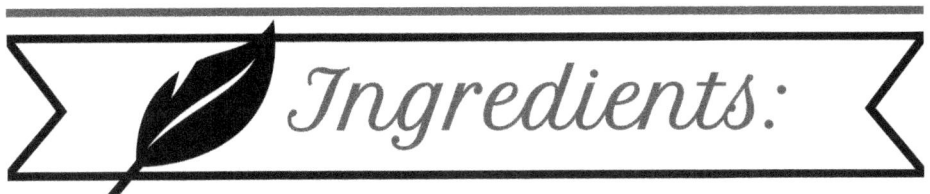

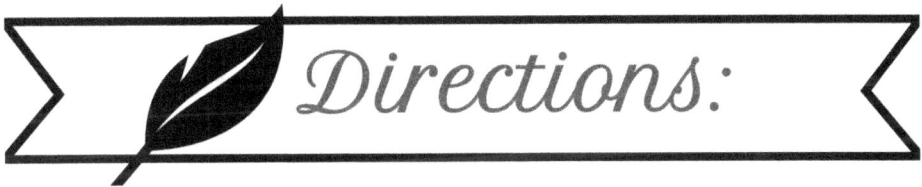

Recipe Name

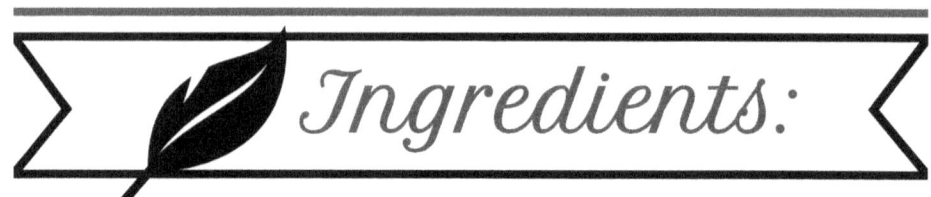

Ingredients:

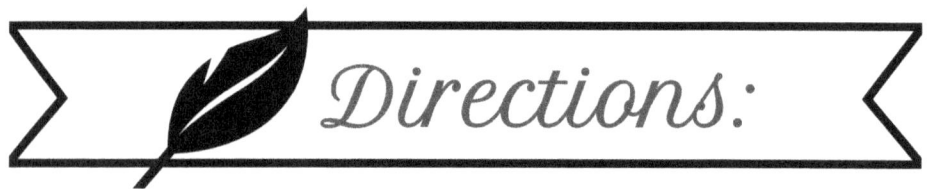

Directions:

Recipe Name

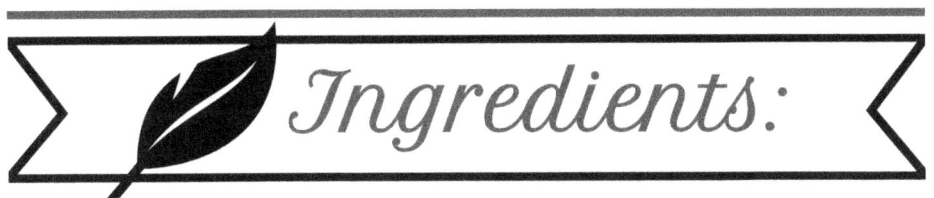

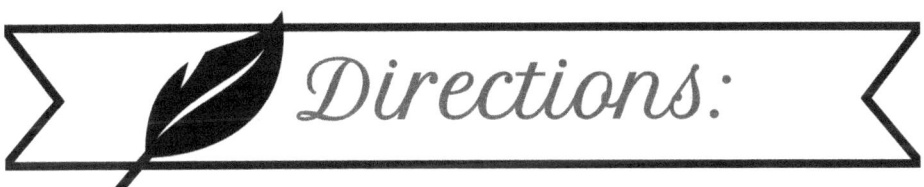

Recipe Name

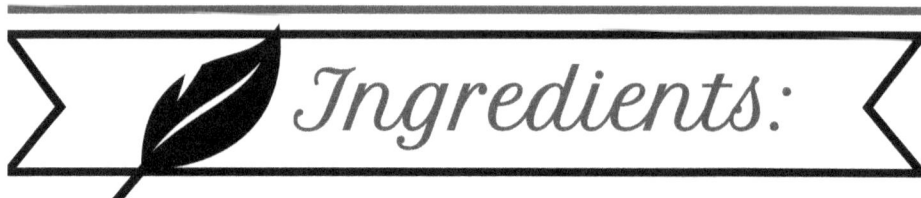

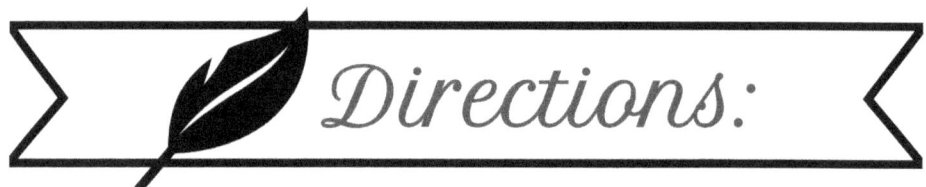

Recipe Name

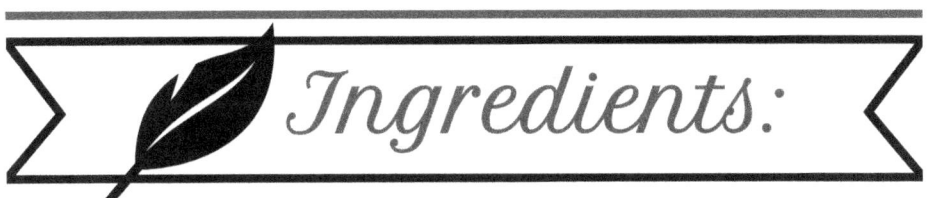

Ingredients:

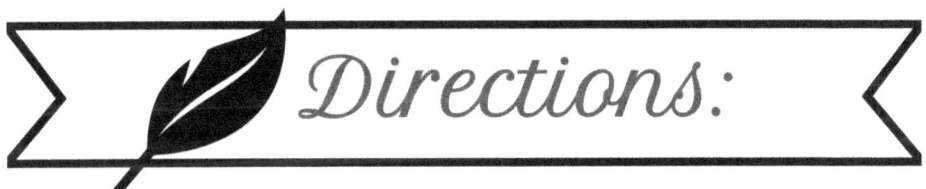

Directions:

Recipe Name

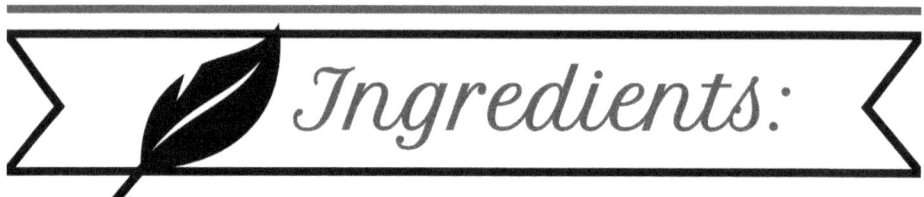

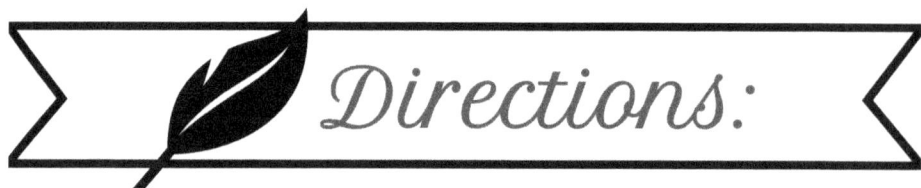

Recipe Name

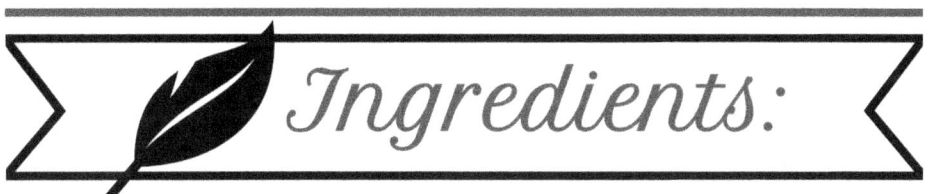

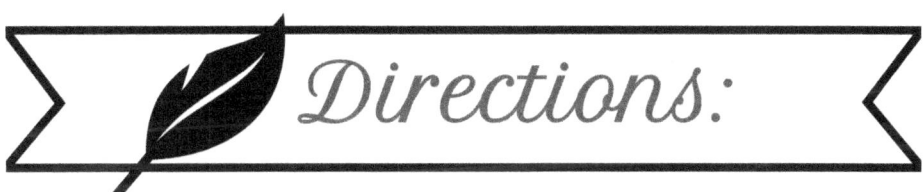

Recipe Name

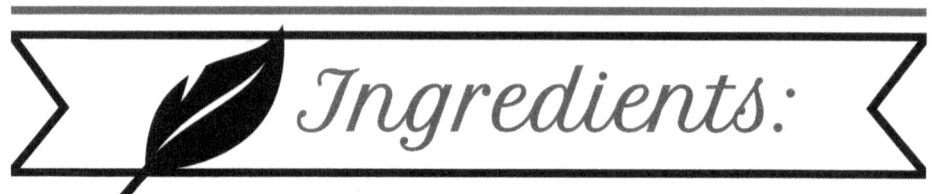

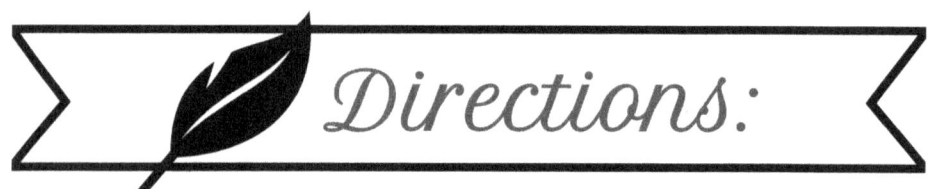

Recipe Name

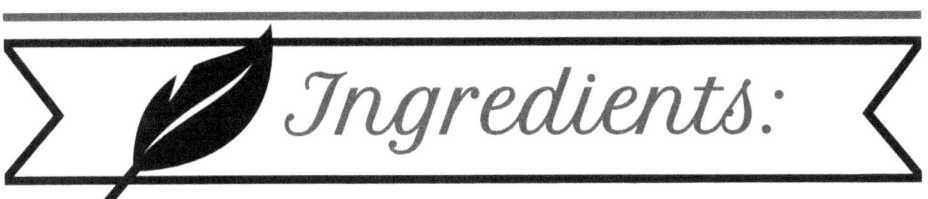

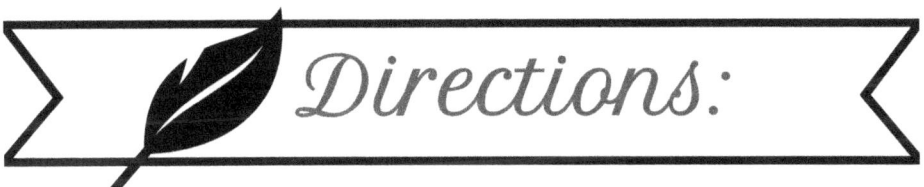

Recipe Name

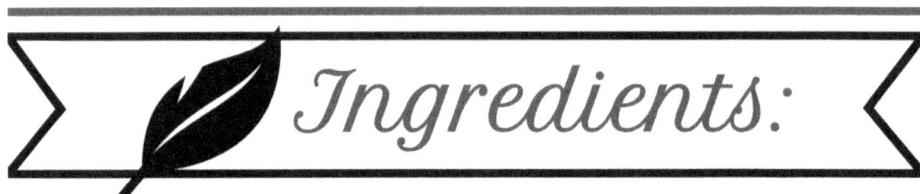

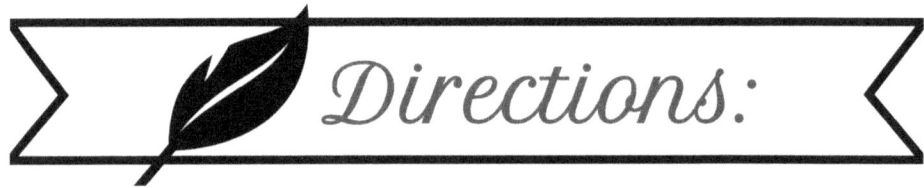

Recipe Name

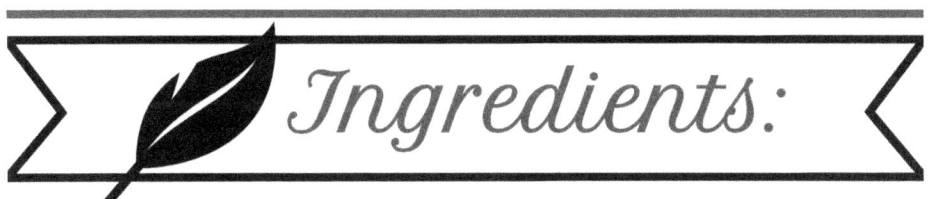

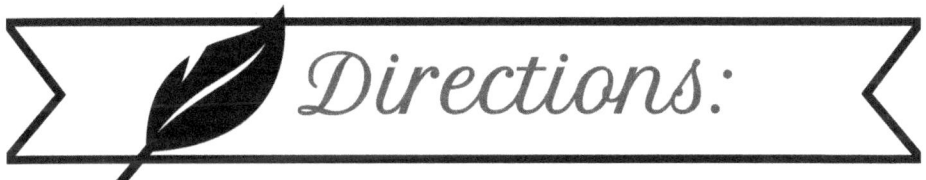

Recipe Name

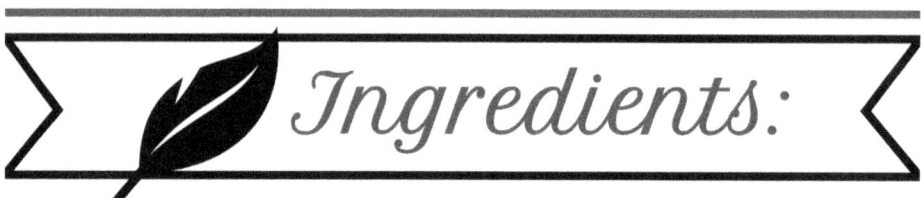

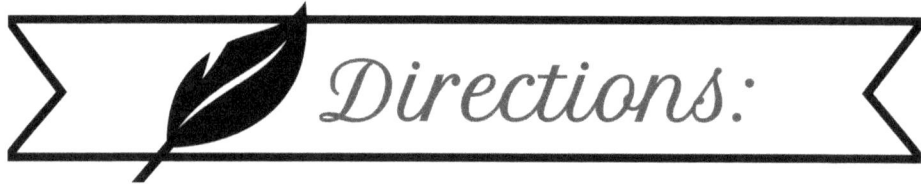

Recipe Name

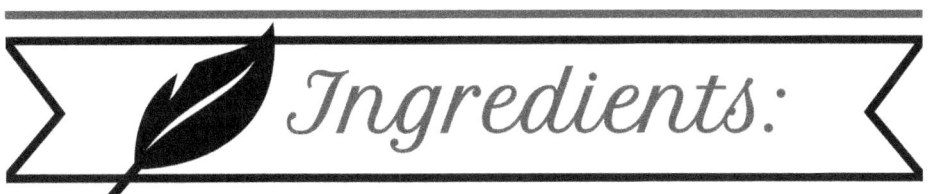

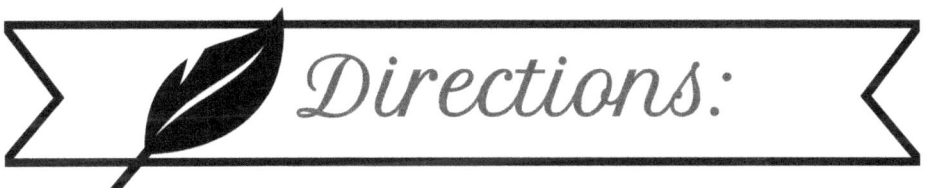

Recipe Name

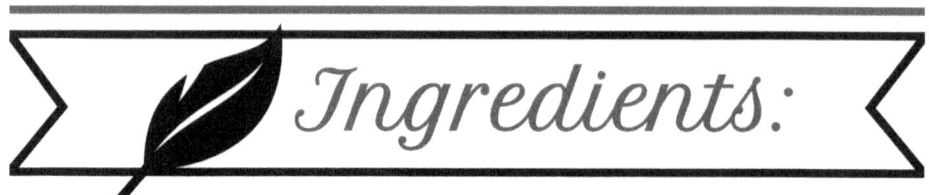

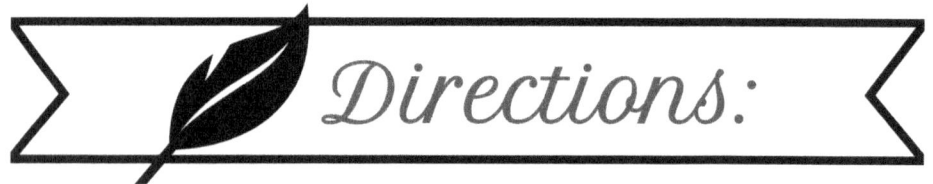

Recipe Name

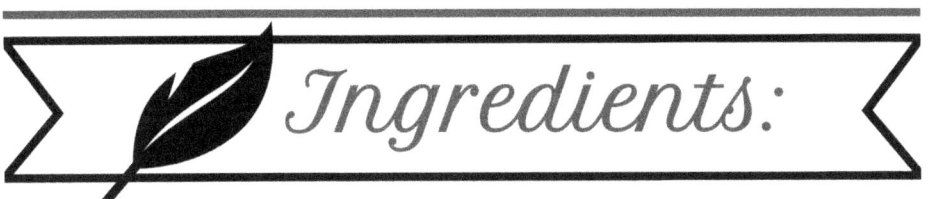

Ingredients:

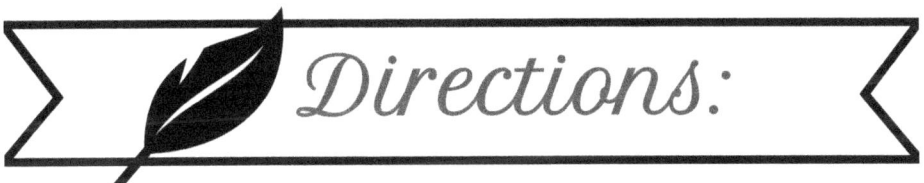

Directions:

Recipe Name

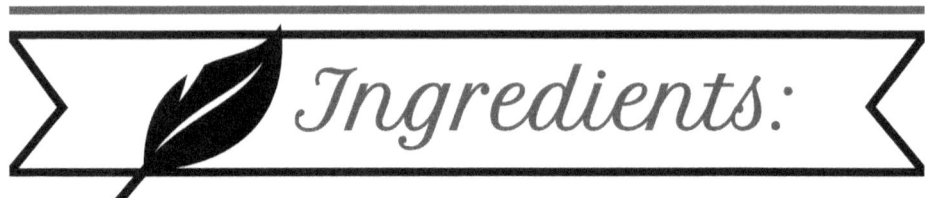

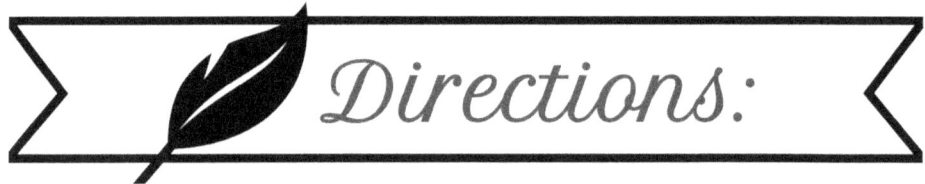

Recipe Name

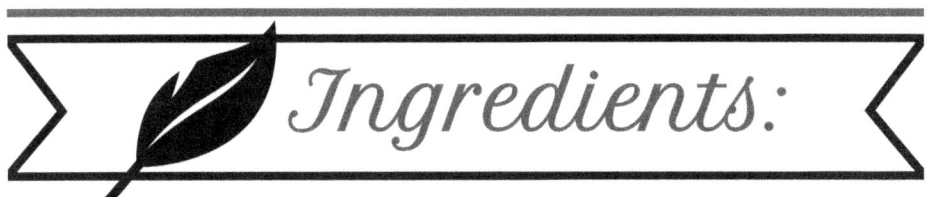

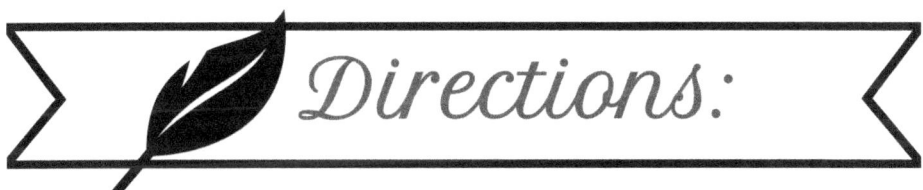

Recipe Name

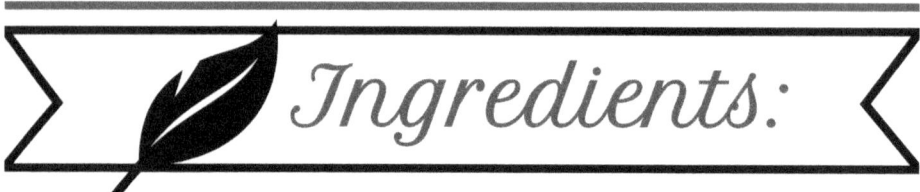

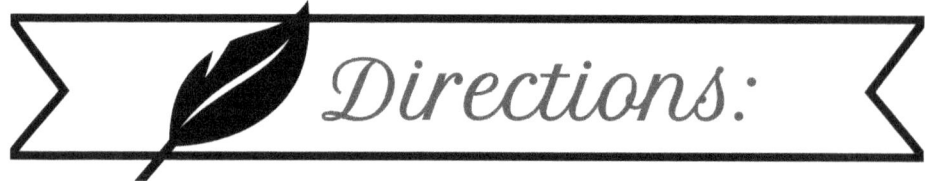

Recipe Name

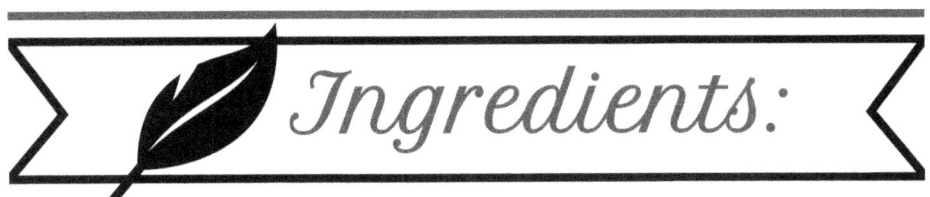

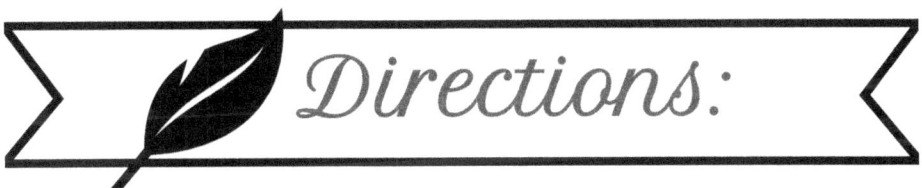

Recipe Name

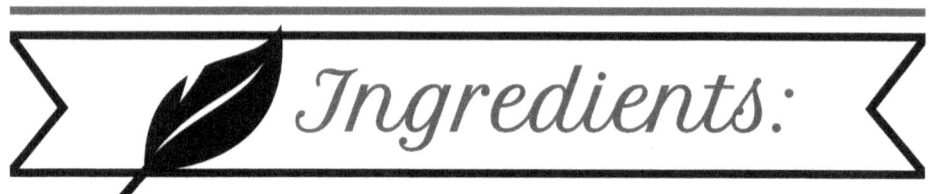

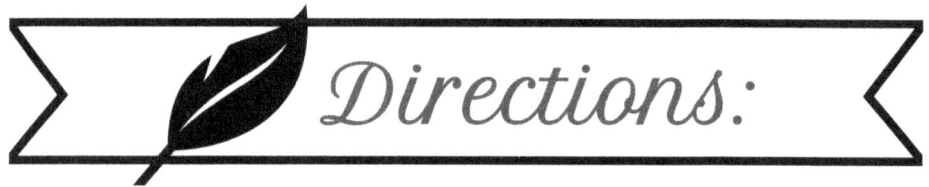

Recipe Name

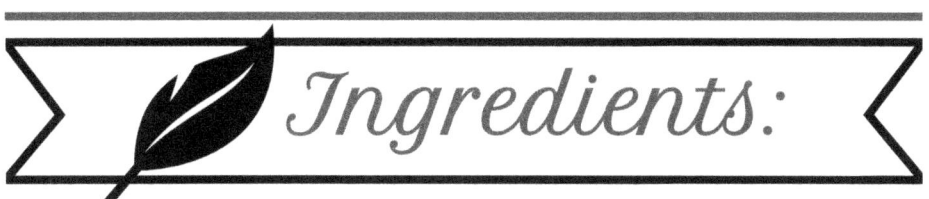

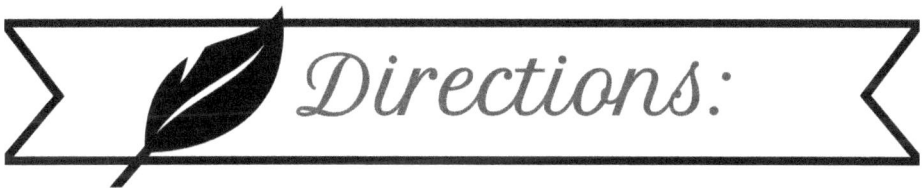

Recipe Name

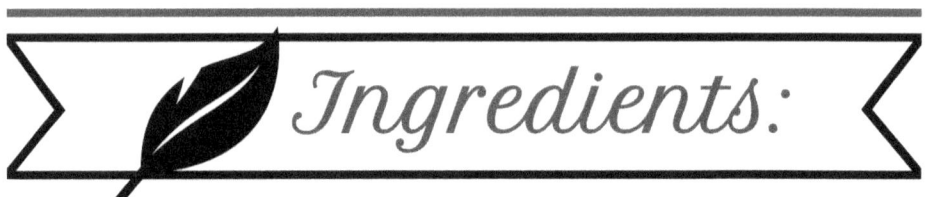

Ingredients:

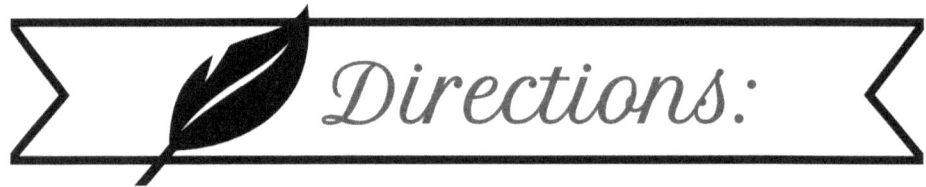

Directions:

Recipe Name

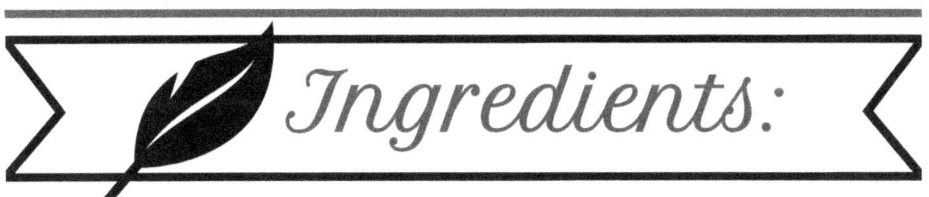

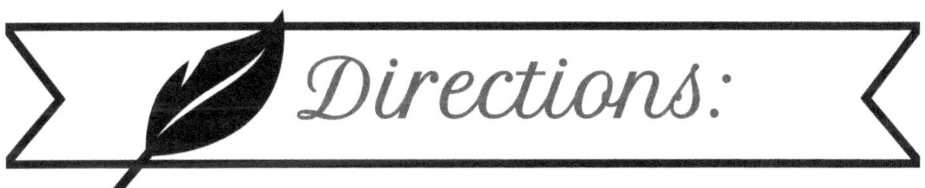

Recipe Name

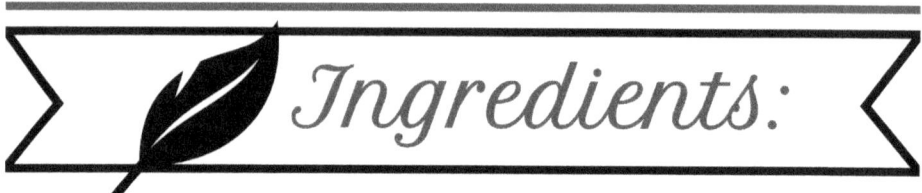

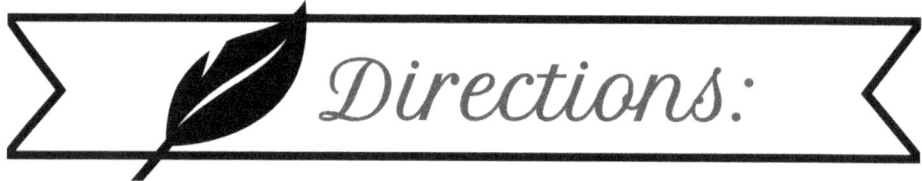

Recipe Name

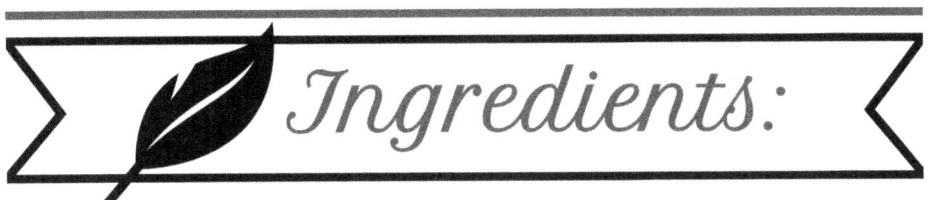

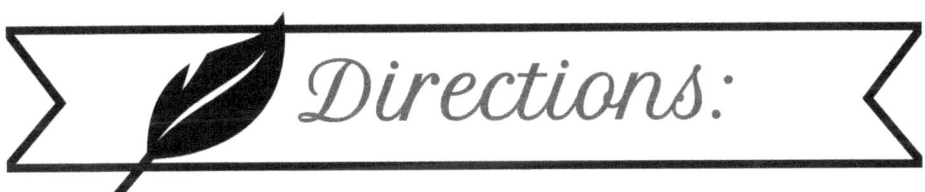

Recipe Name

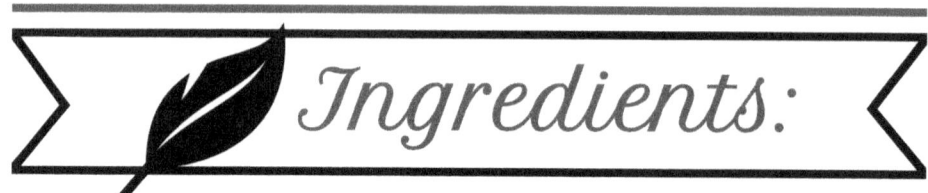

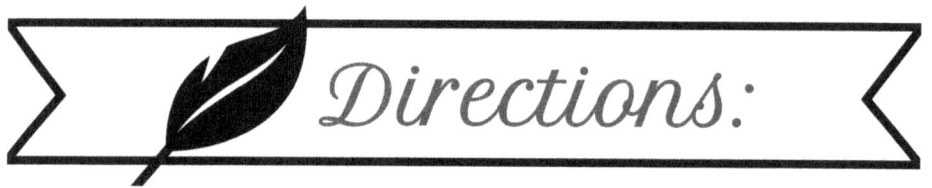

Recipe Name

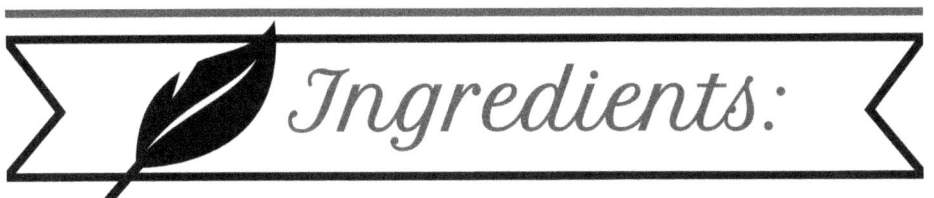

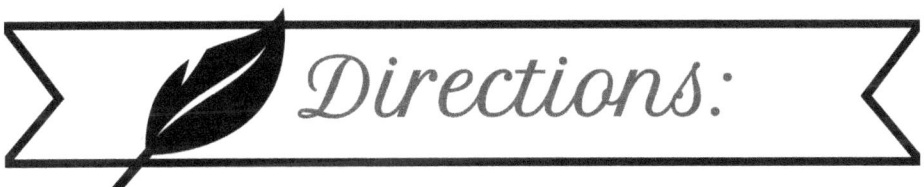

Recipe Name

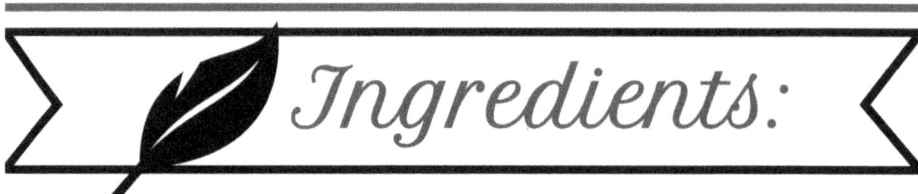

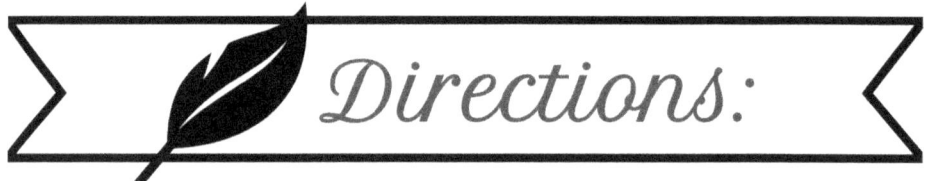

Recipe Name

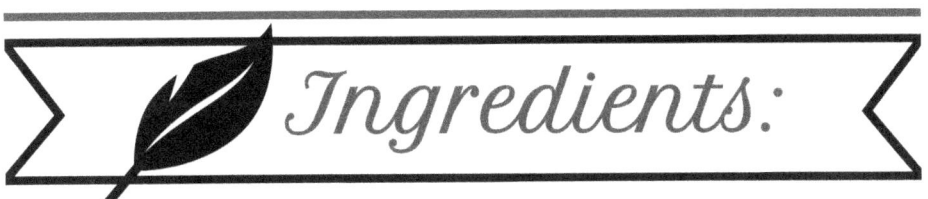

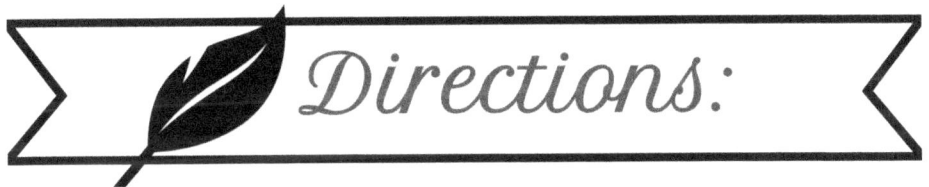

Recipe Name

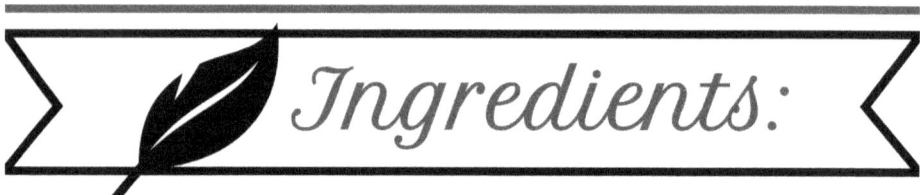

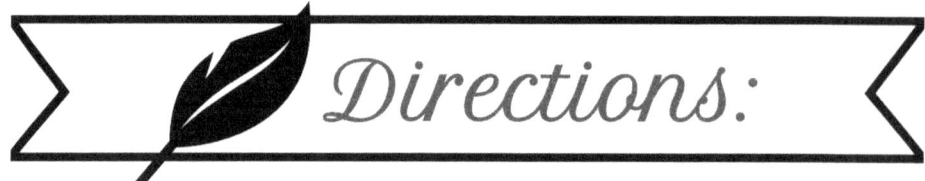

Recipe Name

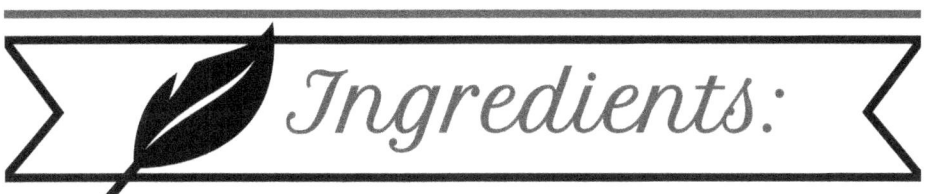

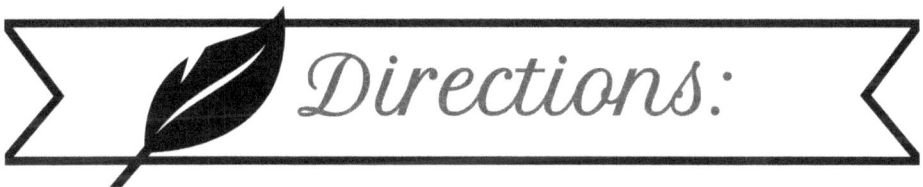

Recipe Name

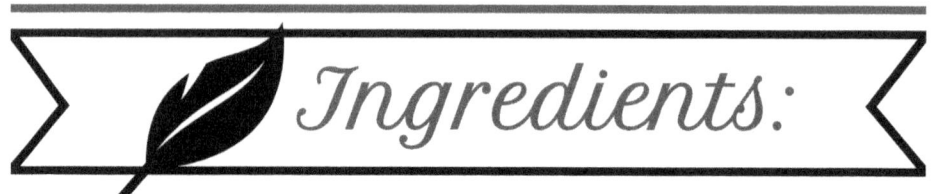

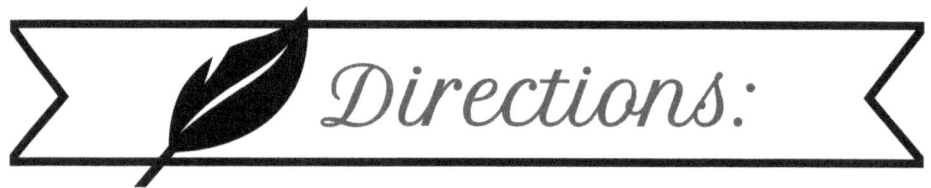

Recipe Name

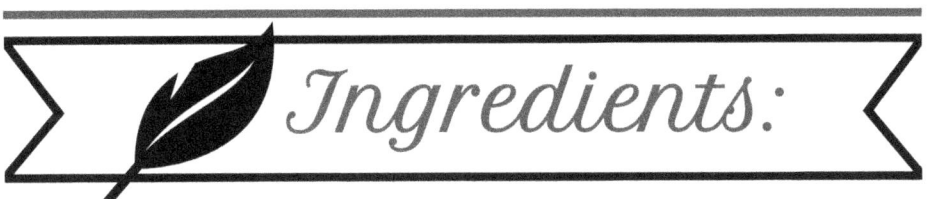

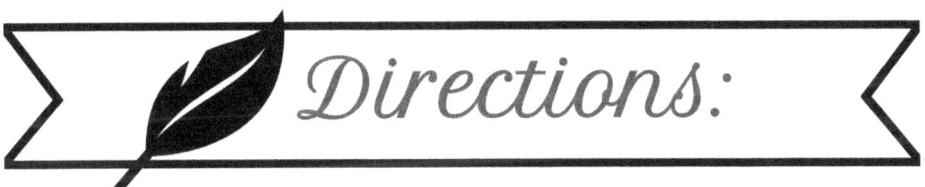

Recipe Name

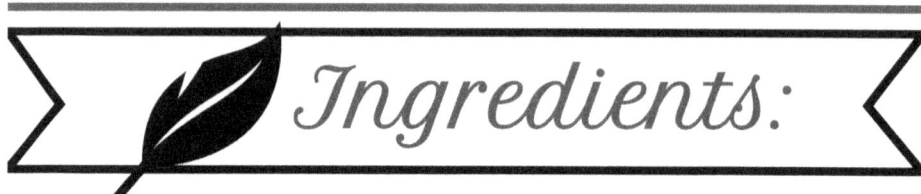

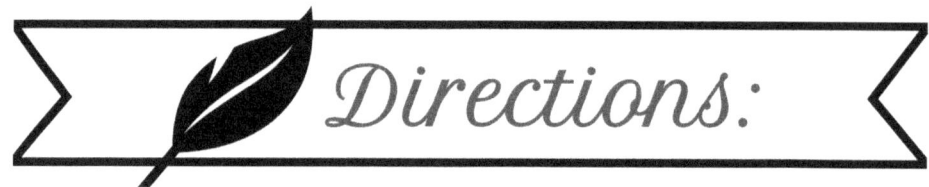

Recipe Name

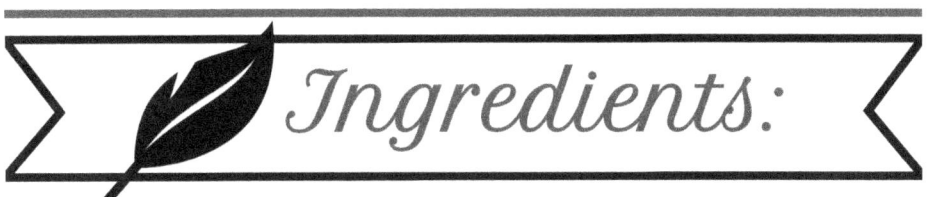

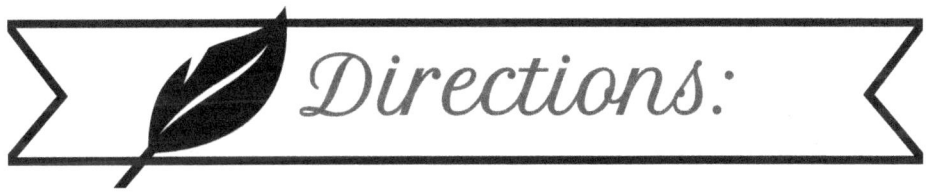

Recipe Name

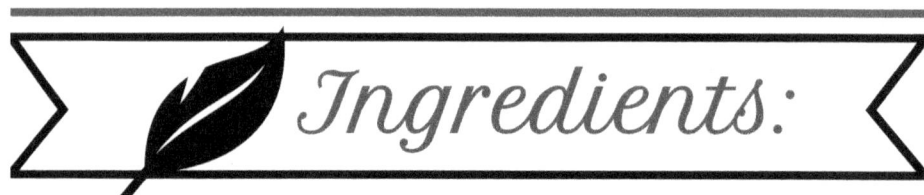

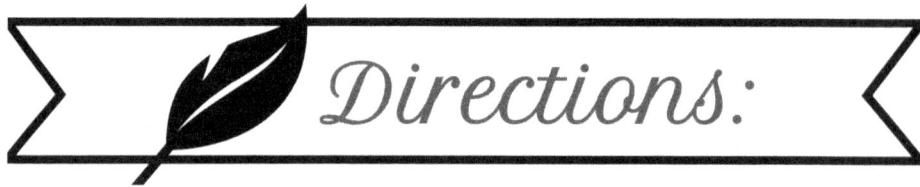

Recipe Name

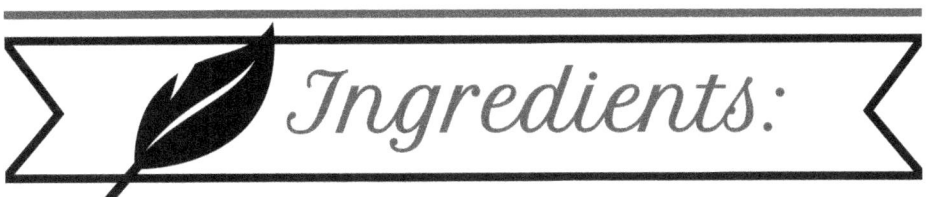

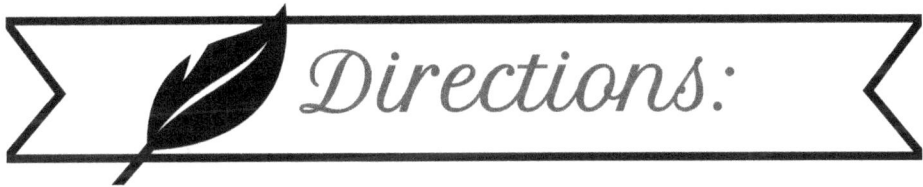

Recipe Name

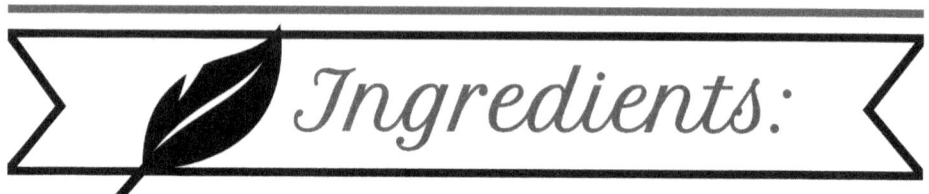

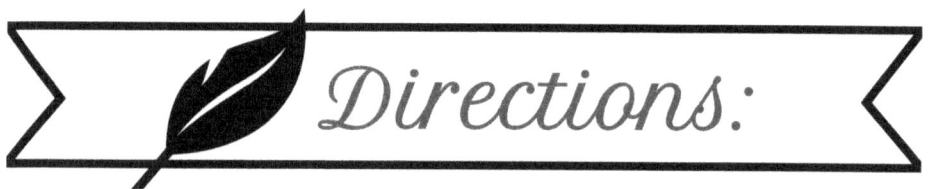

Recipe Name

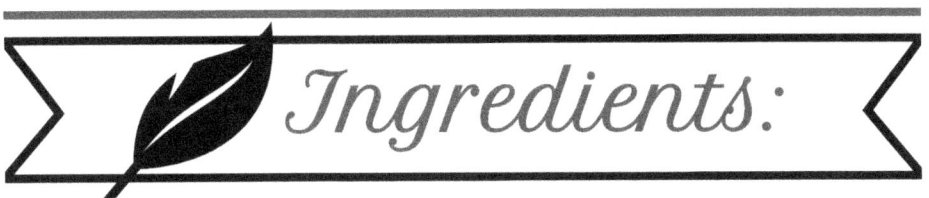

Ingredients:

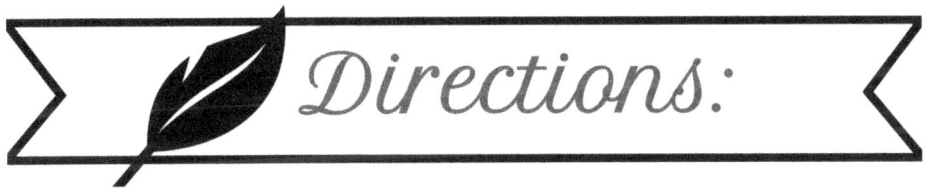

Directions:

Recipe Name

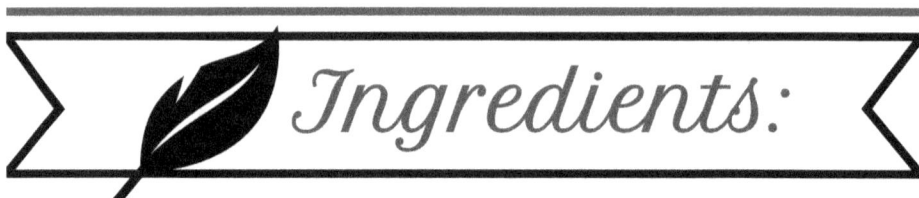

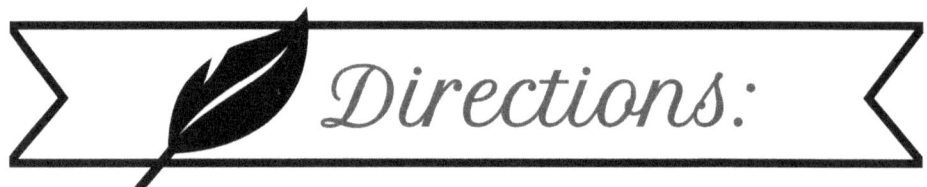

Recipe Name

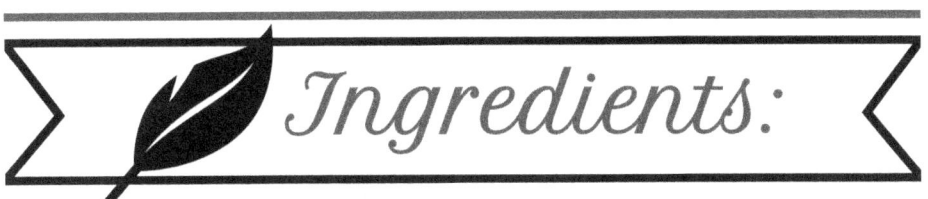

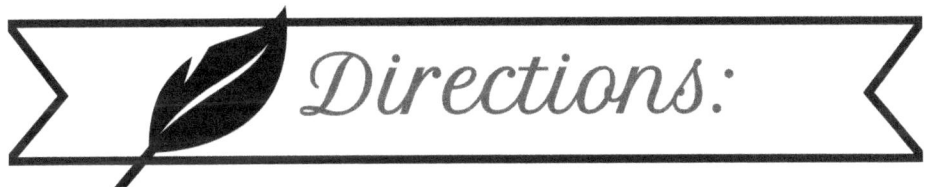

Recipe Name

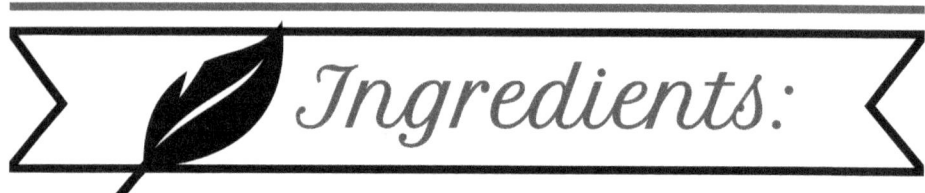

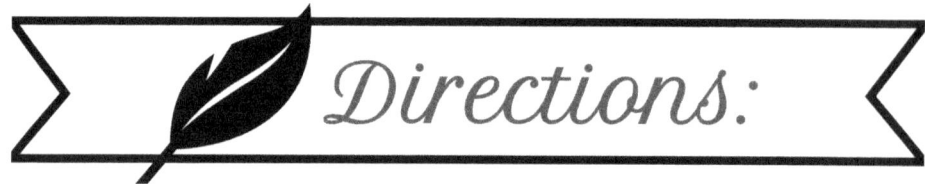

Recipe Name

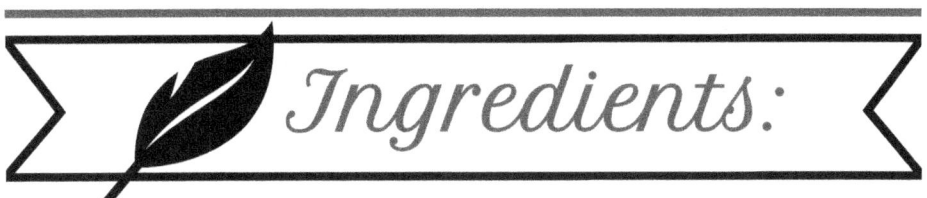

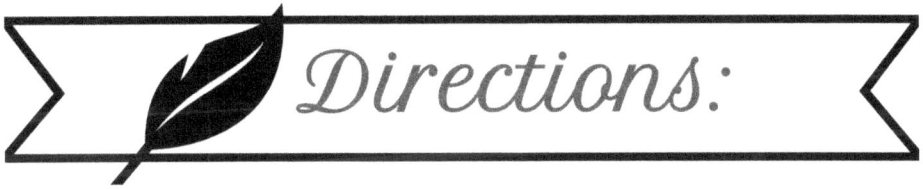

Recipe Name

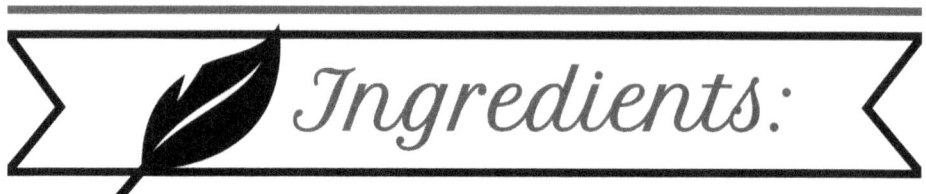

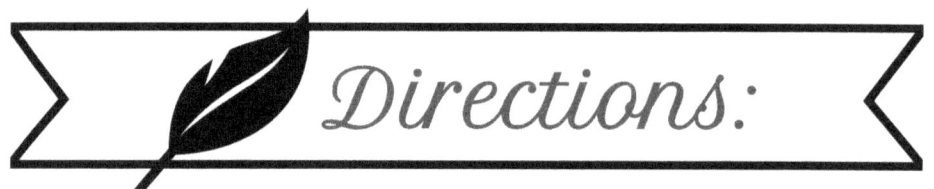

Recipe Name

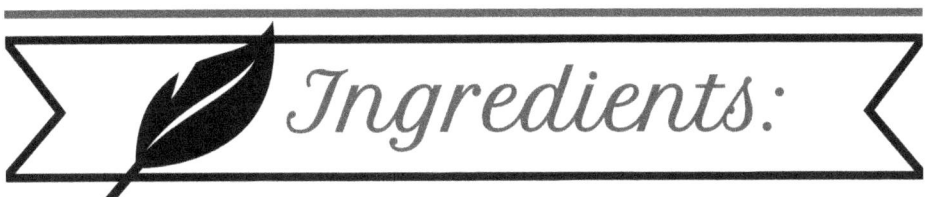

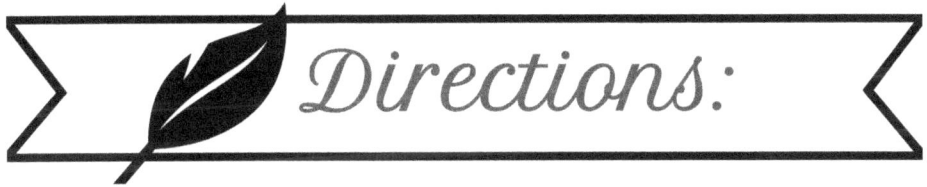

Recipe Name

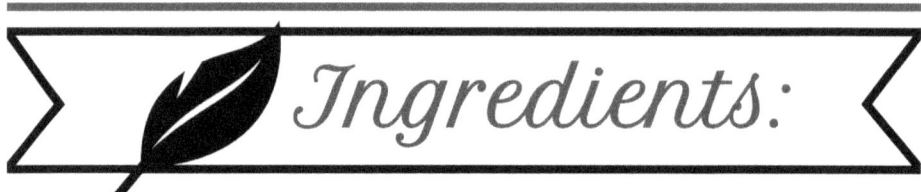

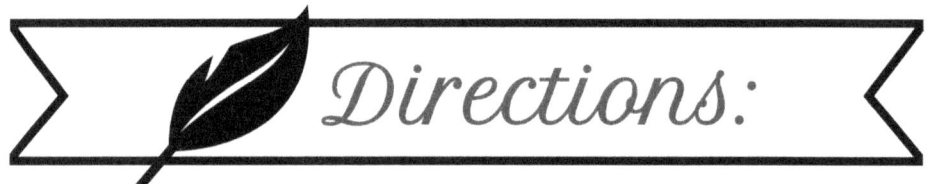

Recipe Name

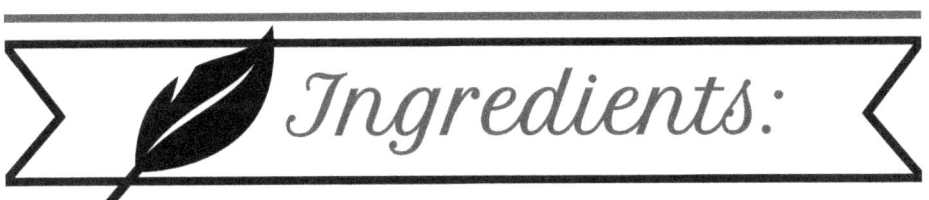

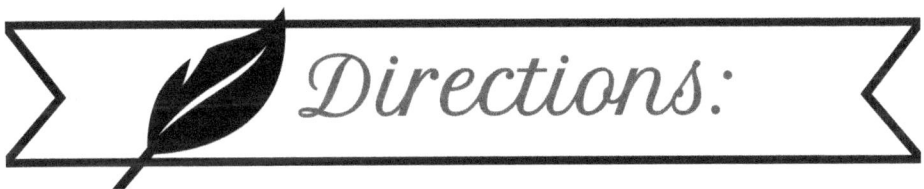

Recipe Name

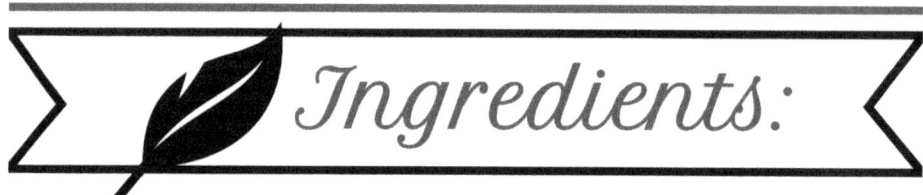

Ingredients:

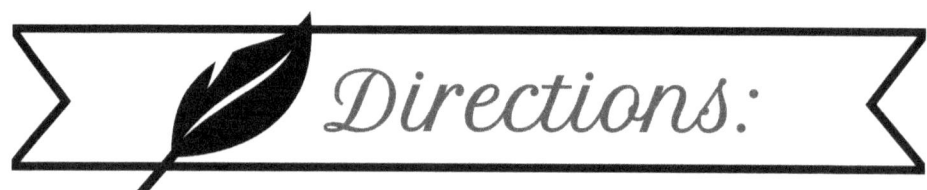

Directions:

Recipe Name

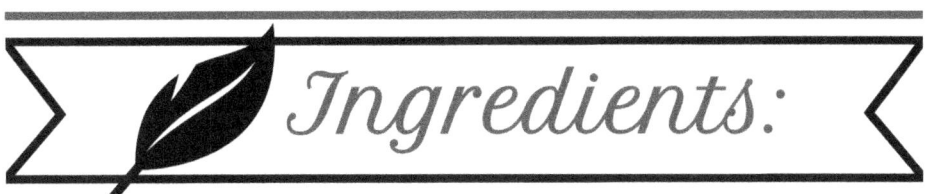

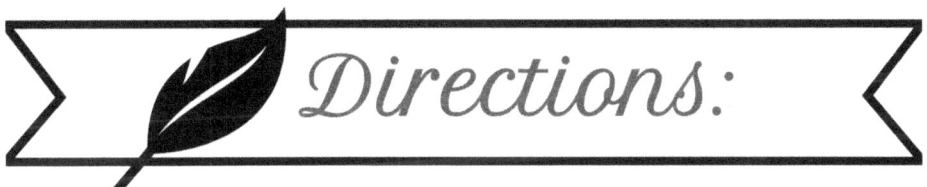

Recipe Name

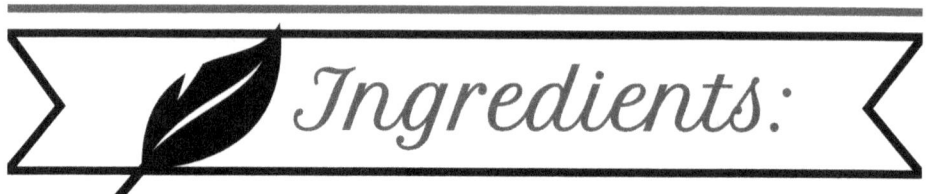

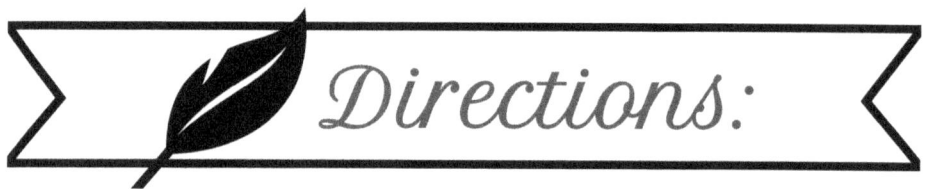

Recipe Name

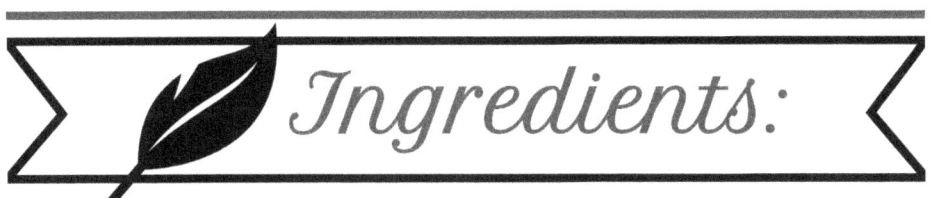

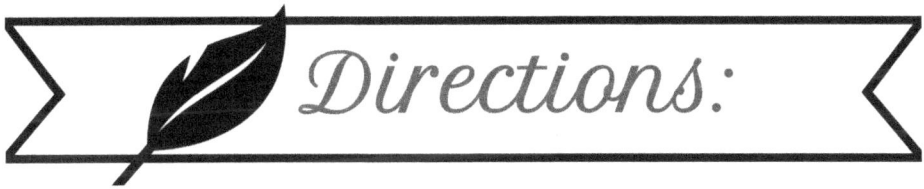

Recipe Name

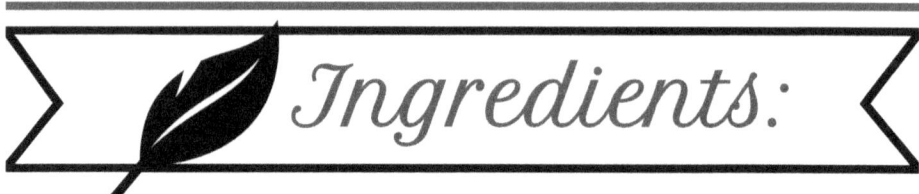

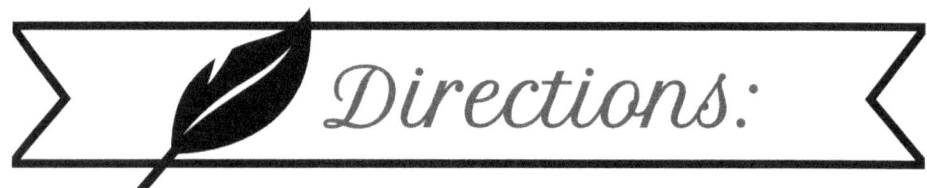

Recipe Name

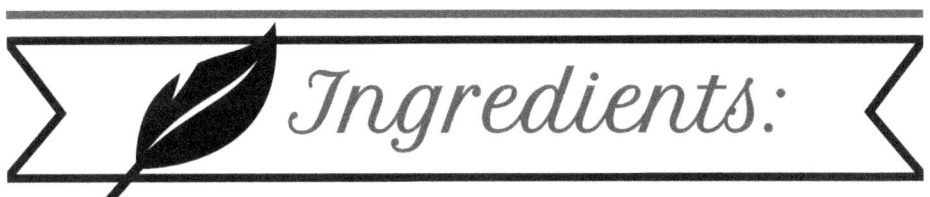

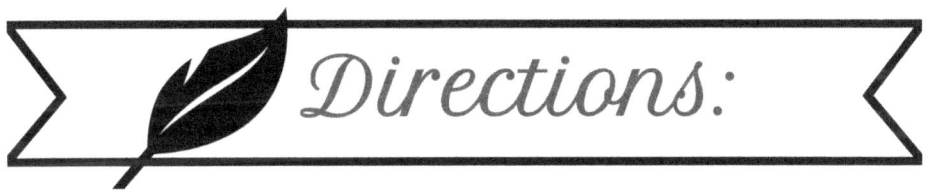

Recipe Name

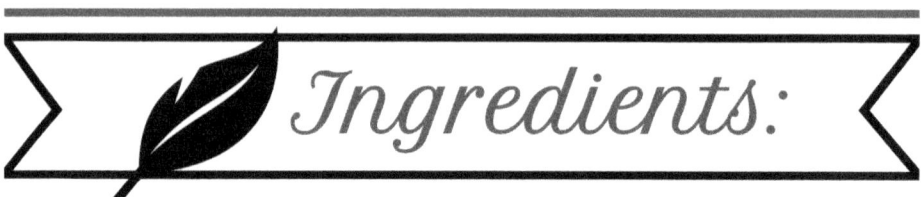

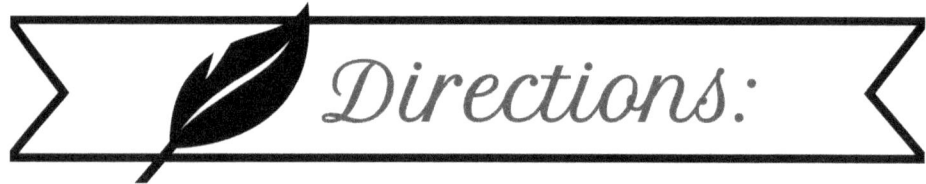

Recipe Name

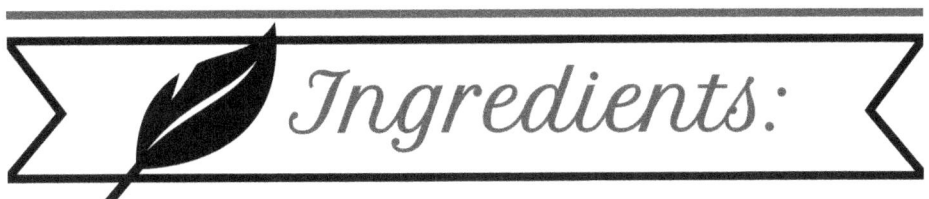

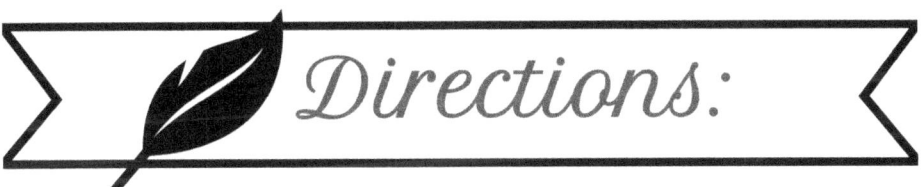

Recipe Name

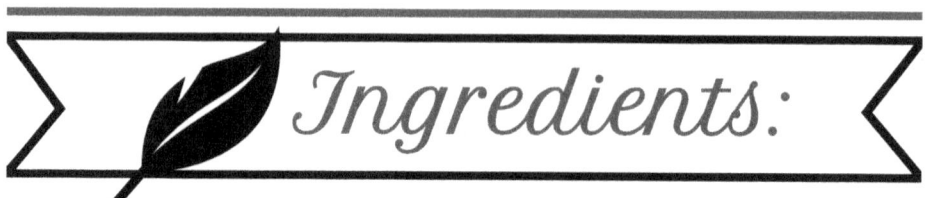

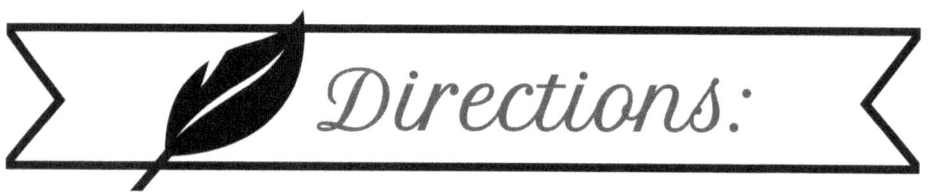

Recipe Name

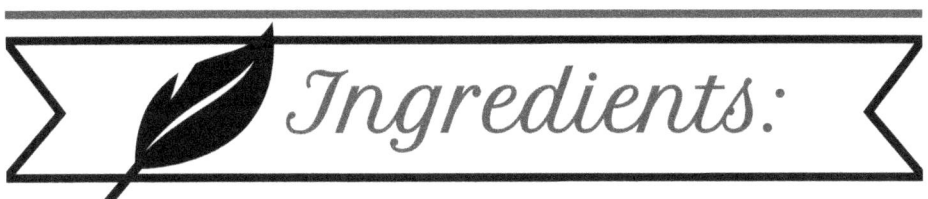

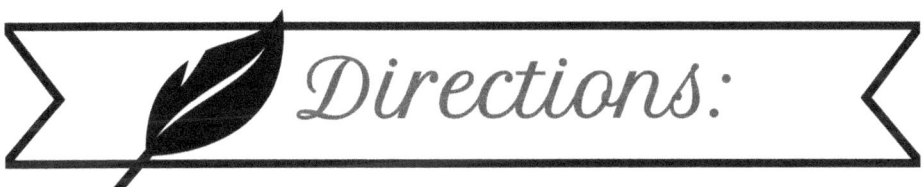

Recipe Name

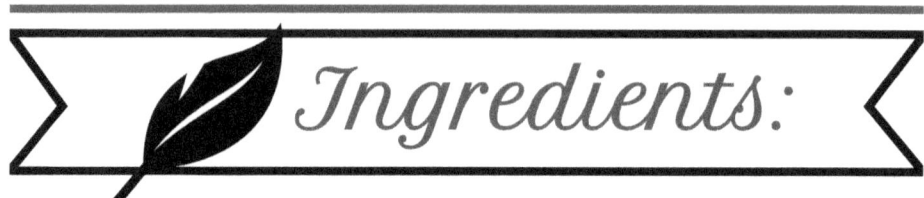

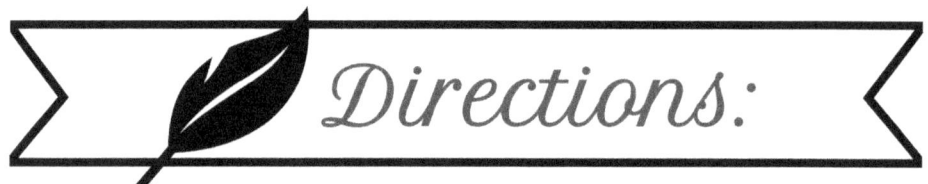

Recipe Name

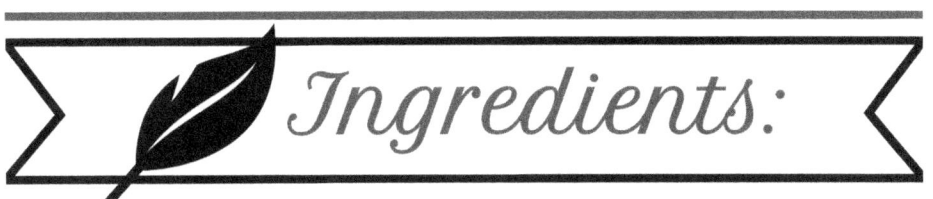

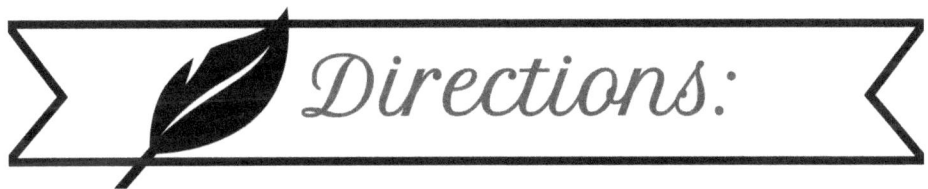

Recipe Name

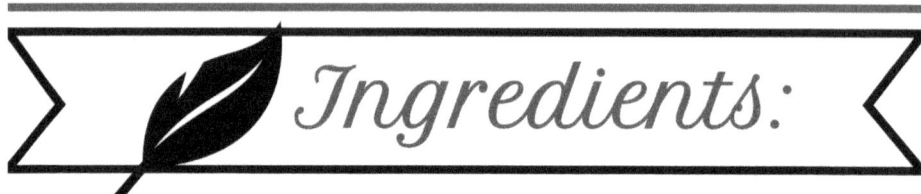

Ingredients:

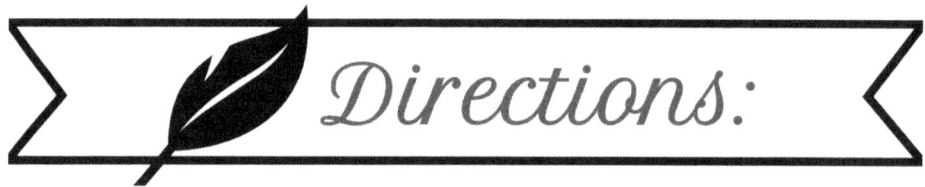

Directions:

Recipe Name

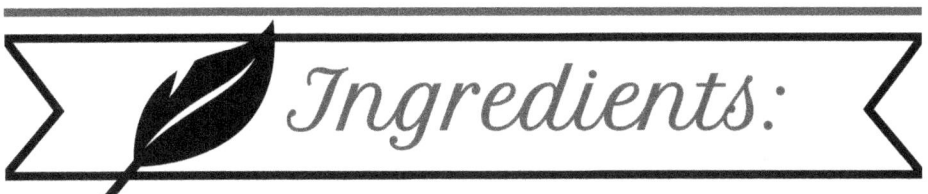

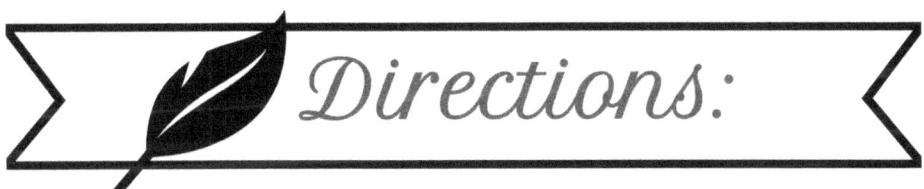

Recipe Name

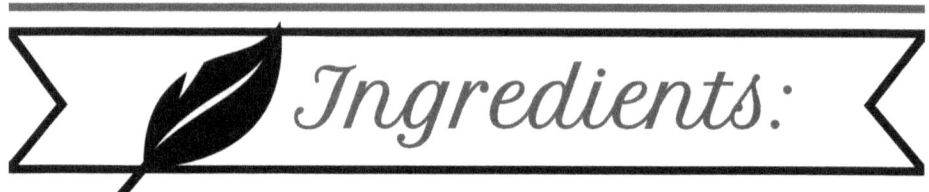

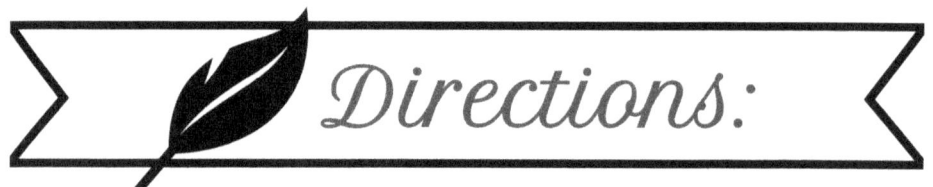

Recipe Name

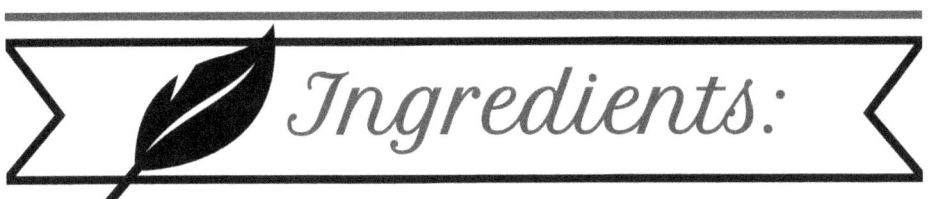

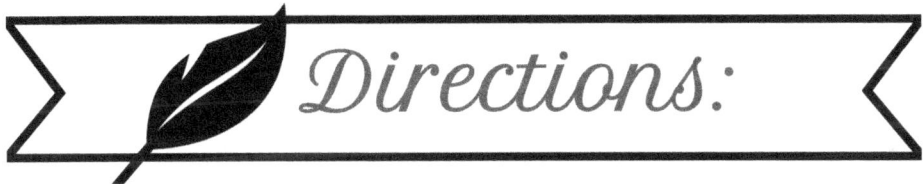

Recipe Name

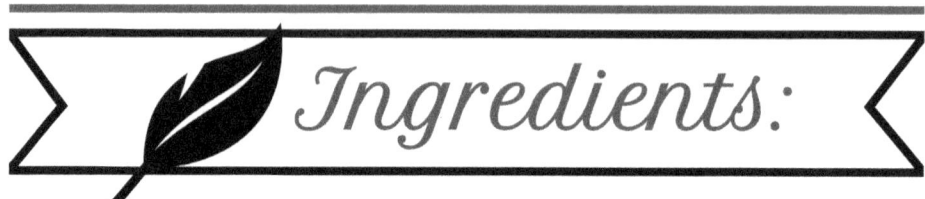

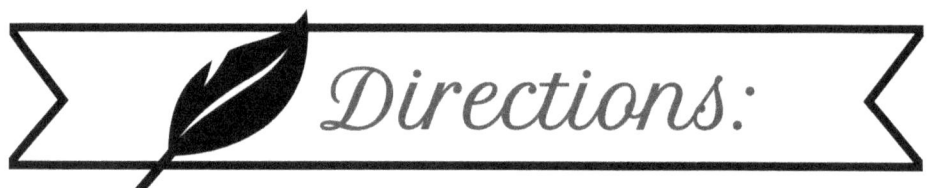

Recipe Name

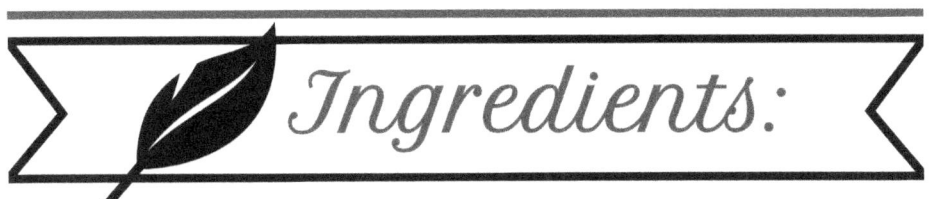

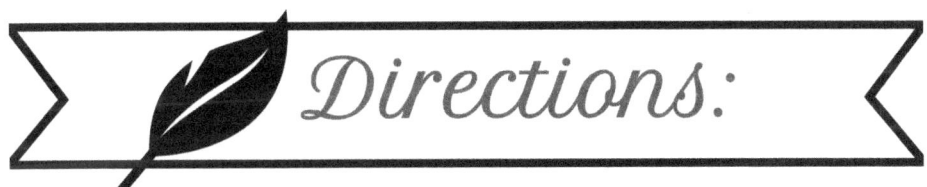

Recipe Name

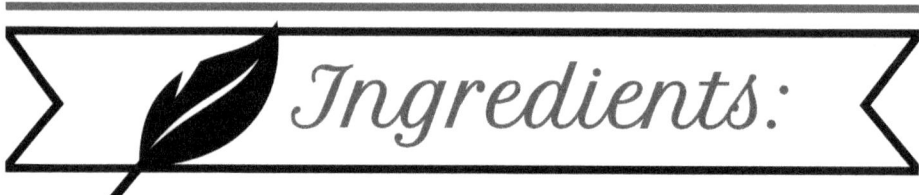

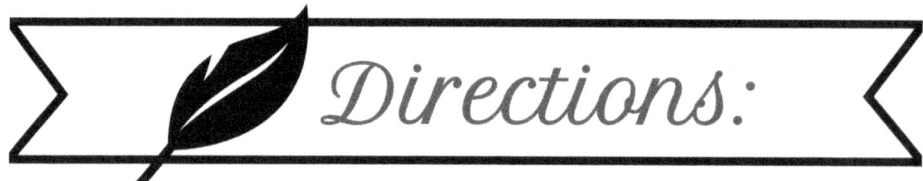

Recipe Name

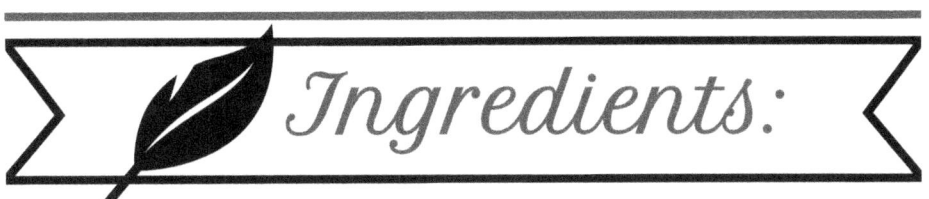

Ingredients:

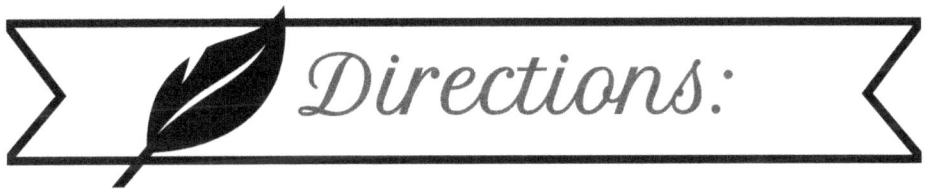

Directions:

Recipe Name

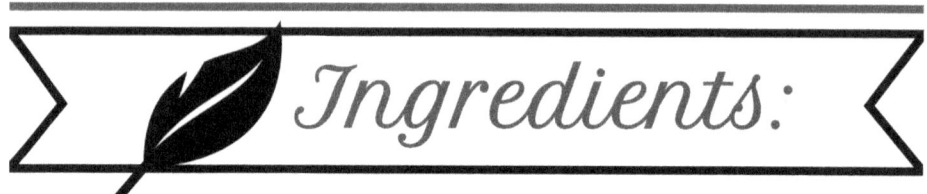

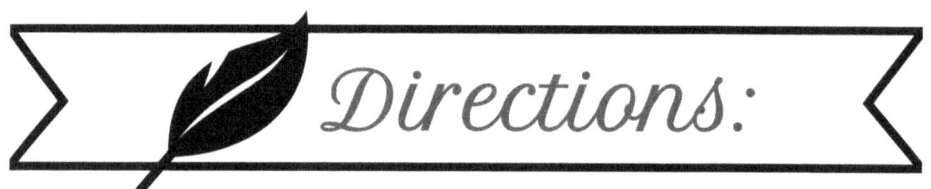

Recipe Name

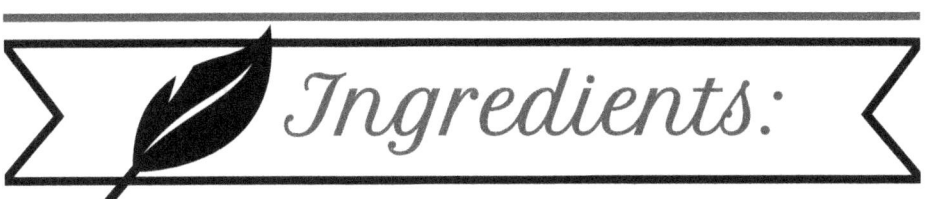

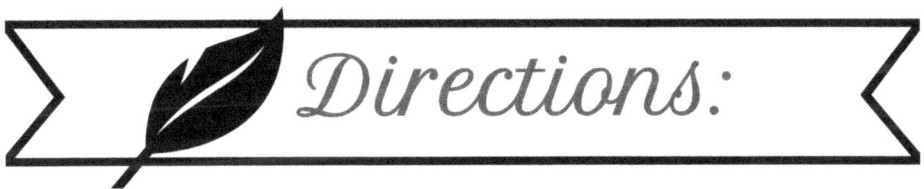

Recipe Name

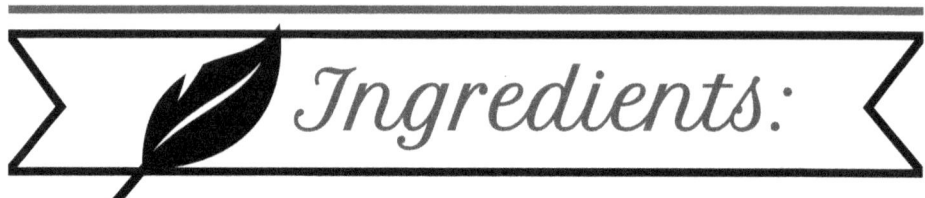

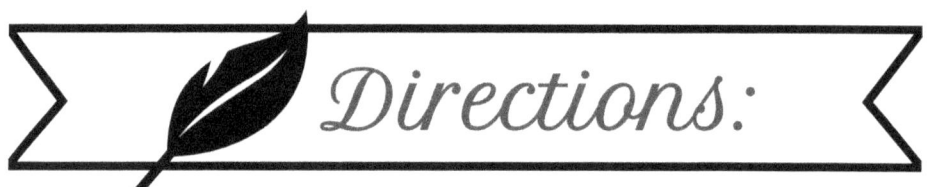

Recipe Name

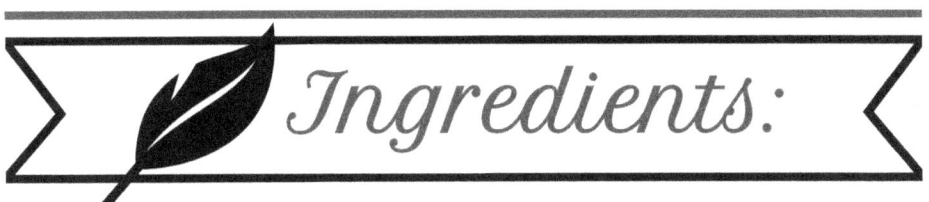

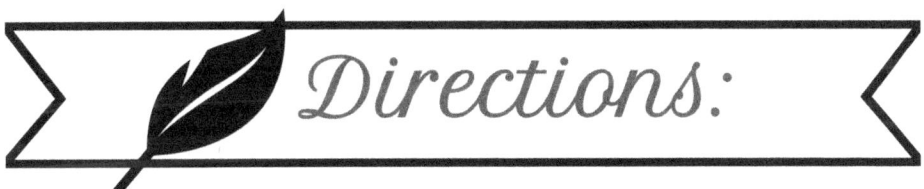

Recipe Name

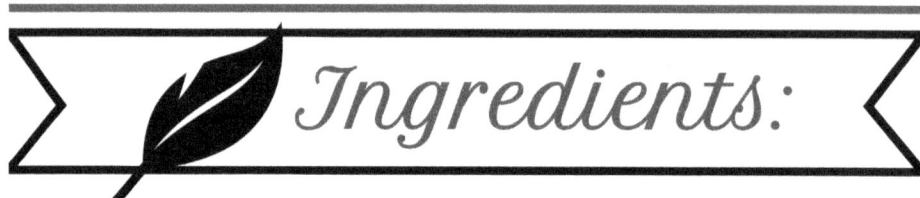

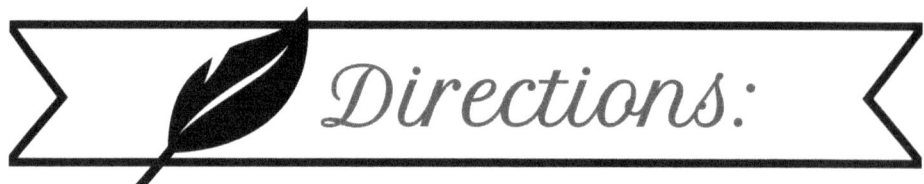

www.ingramcontent.com/pod-product-compliance
Lightning Source LLC
Chambersburg PA
CBHW060416290526
45791CB00002B/779